Faith & Fat Loss

change your body…
transform your soul

by Ron Williams

RTW Publishing International, LLC

Published in Salt Lake City, Utah
by RTW Publishing International, LLC

Cover Design: John Wollinka, Design Corps
Interior Layout and Design: Ryan Lindahl
Photo Credit: Tamara Squires
ISBN -13: 978-0-9817182-2-4
Printed in the United States of America

To God,

who ordained this timely work

and to those who have cried out to Him

for the answer to excess body fat and

acquiring true transformation.

CONTENTS

INTRODUCTION

As one of the most decorated natural bodybuilders in the world, I could have very easily written a book on bodybuilding or fitness, but God has given me a deep love for those who are overweight, obese, and soul wounded. This is not a fitness book – it is a book on health and permanent fat loss.

When it comes to fat loss I am not guessing. As a professor of exercise physiology and nutrition, I scientifically research and teach fat loss. And as a pastor, I believe God wants us to be healthy, so I biblically study health and fat loss and preach it. But more importantly, this is my life and what God has prepared me to do from the time I was born. When the Bible says all things work together for our good this is very evident in my life – from the age of three until now all things, even those that I thought would destroy me, have equipped me to train and coach people to achieve permanent fat loss and true transformation. Faith & Fat Loss is the answer to permanent fat loss, but it is so much more than that. It is a guide to being healthy — physically, mentally, emotionally, and spiritually.

People who are overweight have been stereotyped as being lazy, over-eaters, lacking will-power, and undisciplined. This is a misconception. What I have come to know is many of those who carry excess body fat have been the committed dieters who have disciplined themselves for the short-lived programs that are available. They muster up the will-power, time and time again, to try the next fad that comes along. This is why they have become discouraged and in many cases not willing to try again because they are convinced from experience that it just won't work.

If you have tried any of the fad diets or fat loss programs that have come along and not achieved your fat loss goals you may feel like you have failed, but the truth of the matter is that the diets and programs have failed you. They were not equipped with the necessary fat loss principles, nor did they possess the ability to assist you in losing and keeping the fat off. At most, these programs give you temporary results, which can lead to further discouragement and a damaged metabolism.

If you are struggling with excess body fat you need to know that it's not all your fault. There are many stumbling blocks and hindrances that will make fat loss difficult to obtain. But even worse, the following can actually make losing body fat nearly impossible:

- Excluding God from your fat loss program.
- Not knowing the "root" cause of why you carry excess body fat.
- Lacking the accurate knowledge of how to lose body fat.
- Not understanding the differences between fitness and fat loss.
- Hiding unhealed Soul Wounds.
- Consuming fat loss resistant chemicals and toxins.

Faith & Fat Loss will help you discover the "root" causes of excess body fat and then give you the solutions. By following this program you will learn how to achieve permanent fat loss, true transformation, a deeper intimacy with God, and honor for the power and authenticity of the Bible.

There are many things that will come against you trying to keep you from being successful; including some of the devastating or negative circumstances that have taken place in your life. But it is God's desire to turn these circumstances around for your good {Genesis 50:20}. Regardless of the mishaps, misfortunes, and traumatic events that have taken place in your life remember, *"All things work together for the good to those who love Him and are the called according to His purpose."* Those very things that the adversary tries to use to destroy us and take us down God will use to build depth, character, and compassion, so that we can become the people that He originally intended for us to be.

God is able to make something beautiful out of any situation or circumstance, and my life is a good example of this. Through my experiences, I have developed a personal motto that I continue to live by today, which is that it's not so important how you start, but how you finish.

Most people know me as either an accomplished athlete, a confident speaker, a pastor who preaches the "truth," or as one of the most decorated natural bodybuilders in the world. But this is not where I started. The part of my life that I am going to share with you now is one of the keys that some individuals need to know in order to make permanent fat loss achievable; and it's also one of the reasons Faith & Fat Loss is so different from the many other programs on the market. Through sharing my story, God's intention and my prayer is that it will send a message of hope to those who have been scarred and left with open wounds from past experiences. By understanding my life you will see how God can take an ugly circumstance and make it beautiful, how He can change even your negative thoughts of yourself and make them positive, and take someone who has been deeply wounded and make them whole.

At three years of age I was dropped off at a babysitter's home. My father was supposed to come back, but I ended up spending the next twelve to fourteen years with this family. He left me as a burden on a family of ten that was already doing everything that they could to survive. There was not enough money to provide for the many mouths that needed to be fed and surely not enough for an additional small child. I became an extra body to clothe, and an extra mouth to feed – this later turned into an eating disorder. The couple became the only parental figures that I really knew. I called them Uncle Joe, and Cousin Dorothy.

There would be times when I would overhear Cousin Dorothy talking to my father on the phone telling him, "You need to come and get your son." So, he would come back from time to time and take me for a few days; but since he didn't have a stable home for himself, he would drop me off at different people's houses where the sexual molestation eventually started. The sexual abuse lasted from when I was three until about twelve years old, as I was shuffled between the home I grew up in and the different "babysitters." I had no protection, no refuge, nor anyone that I could confide in to express the pain or the confusion from the variety of abuses. There was no way to stop it and somehow I blamed myself for what was happening. All I knew was that the world was against me and I was completely alone. My circumstances screamed that I could trust no one.

I never felt welcome or like I had a home. I was not part of the family and many times felt like I was an intruder – it was always we have eight kids and him. Christmas was another reiteration of not being wanted. It seemed like everyone had family, but me. As I became involved in sports no one supported me or ever came to any of my games or meets. And the boys, just being boys, would tease me, but because of my unstable mental and emotional state the harsh remarks that were made deepened the wounds that already existed. Things were said like "Go home to your own mom. Oh yeah, we forgot you don't have a mom," or "We found you in the toilet."

Uncle Joe died when I was about eight years old. The last words that I heard him say to Cousin Dorothy were, "Raise this boy, because no one wants him." These words only confirmed what I already felt. And I thought that the only reason Cousin Dorothy took up the burden of raising me was that it was her dying husband's request and not because she loved me. What I knew then was that I was a burden, and I felt like one. I was completely insecure. Always being alone and lonely, not fitting in at home, or school and desperate to understand why no one loved me.

It was my parent's responsibility to raise me, to protect me, to love me, to nourish me, to teach me, and to encourage me. But as a child I did not understand what my mother's life was like or the circumstances of the relationship that she had with my father. I was only aware of the situation that I was left in and what I felt. When I was a small child, I felt a desperate longing for my mother and confusion as to why she didn't come to rescue me. As I grew a little older, it turned into feelings of abandonment and rejection. I blamed her for the physical abuse, the verbal abuse, and the sexual abuse, because I felt if I was with her these people would not be hurting me. I felt the rejection and the abandonment over and over again because I would see her from time to time with my other siblings. I had one older brother and two younger sisters and they were still with my mother. I was the only child who was not wanted, and was not lovable enough for her to keep. This made me feel like there was nothing inside me that was worthy of being loved. This affected every part of me and every single relationship in my life. I became cynical of any love that people tried to give me – I could not give love nor could I receive love. I didn't even know what love was.

Those nine formative years of being shuffled around, abandoned, rejected, and sexually molested left a deep hole in my soul that was meant to keep me from seeing who God wanted me to be. I viewed life through the pain and the tragedy, rather than God's possibilities.

There was a deep hatred inside of me for myself and for humanity. By the age of thirteen, life was so painful I just didn't want it anymore. Suicide felt like my best option and the thought of not being here anymore was actually soothing.

Sports became my family, and the only thing that I had that was worth living for. It was something I was good at it and it made sense to me. If I crossed the line first, I won, there was no second guessing. This is the nature of sports – you either win or you lose. I learned that with people this is just not the case. Every person who should have loved me just didn't. There were so many lies, and people were so unpredictable they said one thing and then did another. With my cup always being half empty the negative in everything always stood out. When someone said they loved me I always wondered what that meant or what they wanted from me. I already knew that I was unlovable, yet these people were saying to me that they loved me. So, subconsciously I drove them away without even knowing it. When they left two things were proven: I was unlovable and that all people are liars.

I was very dangerous because my life meant nothing to me, which made it impossible to care about anyone else's life. Long-term relationships and close relationships were impossible for me. I didn't understand love and my younger years of molestation set a pattern of physical familiarity with the opposite sex, which ended up in my fathering six children at an early age. I had very little parenting as a child, and didn't understand the needs that children had, nor the love that they needed. The only thing that I could do to show any type of love was to provide for them financially because I had nothing emotionally to give. And the best way for me to provide for them was to leave the environment I had grown up in. Now twenty years later, I know that many of the decisions I made were wrong and that my children's lives were affected by bad choices.

To most people I appeared to be fairly normal; partially because through the years I had learned how to function by tucking away and masking the soul wounds, not realizing that they caused me to be relationally dysfunctional.

By the time I was twenty I had competed in four sports on an international level and I was a winner. My quest was to become the best natural bodybuilder in the world, so my life became bodybuilding. I felt that if I became the best in the world the emptiness that I felt inside would finally be filled and I would be satisfied. I remember in 1988 winning my first Mr. Natural Universe title, it was one of the worst days of my life. I felt then that nothing could fill the loneliness, the emptiness, or the hurts that I had suffered throughout my childhood.

At the lowest point in my life, I heard a voice say I am going to take your life. As the sound trembled through me I experienced fear for the first time in my adult life. I heard this voice three different times and was convinced that death was inescapable. Death itself wasn't my fear it was just the thought of being killed that I didn't like.

Being abandoned as a child created a desperation in me not to be alone at night. At night, when I was still and quiet, the pain and hurt of my past many times would be unbearable. In order to medicate myself I would go to a local night club to have a few drinks. The drinking would cover the pain and as a bonus I would take someone home so I wouldn't have to face the night alone. On a particular evening, after I had heard the voice, I asked a woman to go home with me. And after heavy persuasion she agreed. But as the night proceeded I ended up leaving without her. A few days later I saw a news program warning of a young woman who had AIDS that frequented the club that I would go to. She would go to the surrounding hotels with different young men and in the early morning hours she would leave after writing a note on the mirror in lipstick that said, "Welcome to the world of AIDS." She was the same woman I had pressured to go home with me. I knew then that my life was going to end and not knowing where else to go or who to turn to I dropped to my knees. And said, "God if you really love me the way all of those Christians say that you do then help me. If you can take nothing and make something then here is nothing." I, literally, felt God carrying me in his arms for months as he slowly stripped away the outer layers. My healing had began from the many, many soul wounds that controlled my life. For me, healing was like taking layers off of an onion, one painful layer at a time. Forgiveness was the process of letting go and it completely freed me from my pain; not the type of forgiveness that comes from your mouth, but the kind that comes from God that cleanses your heart and soul. This is the process that the Lord has taken me through over the past twenty years. And I am excited about tomorrow because I know that the work God has started He is going to complete. I once looked in the mirror and didn't like who I was, but today I love who I have become.

Are there things in your past that have made you feel discouraged about yourself, your life, your future? Have you tried countless diets and exercise programs, perhaps losing a few pounds but not as many as you'd hoped, or gaining back the weight you lost, plus a few more pounds?

No matter what your past experiences have been—regarding your fat-loss attempts or anything else in your life—you can move beyond those failures and disappointments. By reading and implementing the information in this book, you will equip yourself to lose that unwanted fat, keep it off permanently, and enjoy a lifestyle in which you feel good about yourself—physically, mentally, emotionally, and spiritually.

Are you ready to get started on your new life?

Section I

Change your body... *Transform your soul*

Chapter 1

BEING TRANSFORMED

"Be not conformed to this world, but be ye transformed by the renewing of your mind." —Romans 12:2

A fat-loss craze is sweeping the country. This can be seen by the billions of dollars spent each year on weight-loss programs, products, diets, and gym memberships. If your goal is to decrease body fat, you can find countless methods, solutions, and cures to try. Yet statistics show we are becoming fatter.

The National Institute of Health says that 93 to 97% of all fat-loss and fitness programs fail. More often than not, followers of these programs end up carrying more body fat instead of less.

Evidently, something is missing because what we're doing isn't working.

In order to effectively address the epidemic of being overweight and obese it requires more than a surface answer. Being overweight is only an outward manifestation of a deeper issue. Regardless if you are dealing with misinformation, fat loss resistant toxins, or past hurts the root of the problem needs to be addressed before permanent fat loss can occur. The goal of this book is to inform you concerning what does and does not work, so you can successfully lose body fat permanently.

DON'T BE LIKE THE WORLD

The first part of Romans 12:2 says, *"Be not conformed to this world."* If we are not careful, the world will control our thoughts, our feelings, and our actions.

Television, books, magazines, celebrities, the Internet, and other forms of media bombard us with a maze of information and misinformation. These resources are designed to entice you. They lure you by manipulation, subliminal tactics, and marketing techniques, including attractive colors and music. After "the song and dance" has completed its intended desire by getting you emotionally and physically involved and taking your money, you are left with a feeling of being tricked, scammed, manipulated, and discouraged because you have failed once again in your quest for permanent fat loss. And more often than not, you end up carrying more body fat instead of less. This is what it means to be conformed to this world concerning fat loss.

Being conformed to this world when it comes to fat loss is a natural thing to do simply because many of us have not yet developed an understanding that God is concerned with our health.

Most people think that each part of their life needs to be categorized and administered to separately. When we have a spiritual problem, we bring the situation before our heavenly Father who promises He will meet our needs. When it comes to a medical circumstance, we have been taught to find a doctor. If we are faced with a mental or emotional dilemma, it is natural to seek out psychiatric help. If we are overweight, we consult with a physical-fitness expert.

Categorizing our needs like this is one way in which we have been conformed to this world, when God's desire is to effectively minister to all of our needs.

God wants you to find comfort in the fact that all of your earthly problems have a heavenly answer. If you have a spiritual need be confident, by the prayer of faith, God will grant your request. If you have a medical problem, Scripture says, *"I am the Lord who heals you."* When it comes to emotional problems, the Lord says, *"Come to me and you will find rest for your soul."* For the mind, the Bible tells you to put on the mind of Christ. If your concern is fat loss, turn to the Bible. Throughout Scripture the Lord teaches dietary concepts and the importance of physical movement (exercise). No wonder the Bible says, *"Cast **all** of your cares on Him, for He cares* *for you."* I want to reiterate the word "all"; this unquestionably means every area of your life.

LIFE TRANSFORMATION

In God's wisdom, He directs us in the latter half of Romans 12:2 by telling us, *"Be ye transformed by the renewing of your mind."* Before you can be transformed, there must be a renewing of the mind. The word *"renew"* means to take out the old and apply the new. In this book you will learn the process of genuine transformation, which is the solution to losing body fat permanently.

In order to embrace the physical and spiritual transformation that will result in physical and spiritual fat loss, consider this question: Was it God's original intent for us to be overweight? If your answer to this question is "Yes, I believe His intention is for some of us to be overweight," think about what you are implying. According to some medical specialists, being even ten pounds overweight can cause health problems. If God intended for some of us to carry more body fat than we should, God's desire would be for some of us to become sick and die before our time. I hope you would agree this type of thinking is inconsistent with the loving nature of the God we serve.

True transformation begins with acknowledging your need for God and accepting His plan and purpose concerning your health, longevity, and fat loss.

Spiritual and physical transformation can be compared to a caterpillar that crawls on the ground, and then transforms into a beautiful butterfly that spreads its wings and flies. Once you have fully embraced this thought process you are well on your way to becoming like the butterfly – there is no going back!

Transformation is more than just a change, but you can't be transformed without change. If you only change, you have the ability to go back to the old way of life and to the old you. But once you are transformed, you no longer have the ability to be who or what you once were. Transformation is more than just a change—it is a metamorphosis.

Many secular fitness programs claim they can transform your life, but they only make temporary changes in those who are involved. One of the problems with these programs is that God is left out. Transformation is not just a physical, mental, or emotional change. True transformation can only happen in the presence of a power that is far greater than any man can offer. This can only happen through the power of God.

This is what transformation looks like when it comes to fat loss. Two women who were identical in height and bone structure, each weighing two hundred pounds, decided they wanted to change their physical condition by losing fifty pounds of body fat. Their paths for reaching their fat loss goals were different. One decided to make a change by using the latest secular fad fat-loss program. She changed and lost fifty pounds! But because she only made a change, she quickly gained back the fifty pounds, plus an additional ten.

The second woman had a different mind-set and sought God's help for more than just a change. Her desire was true transformation. She was sick and tired of just change, and wanted permanent fat loss. She searched in Scripture and found the necessary tools to decrease body fat permanently and God's promises concerning every area of her life. Like Second Corinthians 5:17 says, *"If anyone is in Christ, he is a new creation; the old has gone, the new has come."* Old things have passed away and are gone. Her obesity was an old thing. She became something new. She lost the fifty pounds she sought to shed, and kept it off, permanently maintaining her fat-loss goal. This was a metamorphic experience or true transformation. She no longer had the ability to go back to what she once was.

When it comes to fat loss, we cannot settle for temporary change. We need a life transformation for lasting results.

Transformation takes place when you turn your life over to God and yield to His instruction. When something is broken inside you, God is the only one who can reach into the depths of your soul, destroy the yoke of bondage, and fix that which is broken. God's desire is that each of us would be transformed (Romans 12:2).

GOD: THE ANSWER TO PERMANENT FAT LOSS

God wants to provide for **all** areas of your life. In First Peter 5:7, the Bible states that the Lord wants you to *"Cast **all** of your cares upon Him, for He careth for you."* God is not merely suggesting that you cast your cares on Him. This is God's plan. He wants to meet **all** of your needs. In many areas of life, you will encounter circumstances and problems that He alone has the answer to. If you are concerned (or care) about being overweight, take the time to involve God in your plan for fat loss.

God's way to permanent fat loss is 100 percent effective. He will supply the knowledge, and give you the ability and the discipline to complete your spiritual and physical transformation. Your part is simply to accept the knowledge and the ability, and to apply the discipline that God has given you.

THE BIBLE: THE BASIS OF THE PLAN

You may feel you've tried every diet on the planet. You searched multiple resources, consulted numerous so-called fat-loss experts. But have you looked in God's Word? The Bible is our Owner's Manual. Throughout Scripture, God has revealed timeless dietary concepts, supported by true science, that produce permanent fat-loss success.

The Bible tells us not to put our confidence in man's efforts alone {Philippians 3:3}. I am not suggesting that human effort has no merit, but I am suggesting you put your confidence in something that knows no failure: God.

Ecclesiastes 1:9-10 teaches us, *"There is nothing new under the sun. Is there anything of which one can say, "Look! This is something new"? It was here already, long ago; it was here before our time."* True science is only the discovery of God's natural laws and principles and always agrees with Scripture. This means that the answers or truths we are seeking have always been there, they just need to be revealed or discovered. Every situation and every circumstance that deserves an answer, including nutrition and permanent fat loss, is found in God's Word.

Hopeless or Hopeful?

When you come to the realization something is wrong in your life and acknowledge that you can't fix it, you may feel a sense of hopelessness. Don't let that feeling cause you to give up. Instead, allow yourself to embrace God's help. This is the starting point for God to accomplish what only He is capable of doing.

In Jeremiah 18:4-6, God revealed to His prophet the concept of transformation through an illustration. *"The jar he was making did not turn out as he had hoped, so he crushed it into a lump of clay again and started over. Then the Lord gave me this message: O Israel, can I not do to you as this potter has done to his clay? As the clay is in the potter's hand, so are you in my hand"* (NLT).

Make the Commitment Today

I would like to encourage you to make a prayerful commitment to allow God to transform your body and your life. I have prayed for your success. Jesus died for your success. God gave Heavens best for your success. The only one left in this equation is you. If you accept this worthy endeavor, you will not be disappointed.

As children grow, they go through growing pains. As we experience transformation, our spiritual growth will cause spiritual growing pains. You will face deterrents, such as negative emotions and fears that will try to discourage you from completing this process. You may experience discomfort, anger, loneliness, withdrawals, sabotage, and disappointment. Even though transformation may not come easy, it will be one of the most life-changing experiences you will ever have. The rewards are monumental. You will look better, feel better, and become more productive. Your life will be extended, which will increase your capacity to give to others. Most important, your spiritual transformation will transcend throughout eternity.

My Prayer

In writing this book, I have prayed to God on your behalf. Here is my prayer for you today:

Lord God,

Your Word says, "Look to the hills from whence cometh my help. My help comes from the Lord." Lord, I am asking You today for Your help. The people reading this book may be struggling with depression, past abuses, soul wounds, being overweight or obese, and suffering from obesity-related diseases. I cannot sit idly by and allow them to continue to suffer when I know you not only have the answer, but you are the answer. Lord God, be the answer to the people reading this book right now. Be a very present help in this time of their need. I pray the gifts will be stirred up. I pray discipline will be transferred. I pray for healing to occur. Lord, I pray that You would make Yourself more real in their lives than they could ever imagine. I give You praise, glory, and honor. I thank You in advance for the victory of the individuals who are reading this prayer right now, that their lives would be transformed, physically and spiritually. In Jesus' name. Amen.

If you agree with this prayer, I want you to say out loud:

"I receive the words of this prayer for my physical and spiritual life. I am making a personal declaration of transformation. In Jesus' name. Amen."

Implement the Truths

The Scriptures contain the guidelines, parameters, and requirements for our spiritual and physical transformation. Through the pages of this book, you will learn the spiritual, physical, scientific, and historic truths concerning transformation and permanent, healthy fat loss.

By implementing the following truths, your battle with excess body fat will finally be won:

❖ **Accurate Knowledge** – The Faith & Fat Loss program is based on biblical principles that true science agrees with. This program has the physical and spiritual answers to address the problem of being overweight and obese and will ultimately lead you to true transformation.

❖ **Soul Surviving** – This is the process for overcoming soul wounds in order to be healed physically, mentally, emotionally, and spiritually.

❖ **The Power of 21** – The first 21 days of the Faith & Fat Loss program is a period of physical and spiritual detoxification and a "Jump Start" to your permanent fat loss. It includes; twenty-one days of nutrition, twenty-one days of Scripture, twenty-one days of exercise, and twenty-one days of prayer.

❖ **The Eating Plan** – The diet and nutrition portion of this program is based on practical biblical and scientific principles that can be used in the average individual's everyday life.

❖ **The Spiritual Eating Plan (The Word)** – Scripture is the source of our faith and says that nothing is impossible to them who believe. We draw from God's Word for comfort, discipline, strength, faith, encouragement, and healing to complete our life transformation—physically and spiritually.

❖ **Exercise** – Exercise is a vital part of the Faith & Fat Loss program. It shapes, sculpts, and strengthens the body; increases metabolism; changes your moods by release of serotonin and endorphins; increases energy; and much more.

❖ **Spiritual Exercise (Prayer)** – Prayer is the medium God chose for us to communicate with Him. This is how we develop our relationship with Him. Through prayer He reveals who we are created to be and what we are supposed to accomplish in every area of our life, including fat loss.

❖ **Supplementation** – Supplementation means "in addition to," not in place of. In order to achieve optimal health and fat loss, proper supplementation is necessary.

Section II

Discovering "The Root"

Chapter 2

THE DANDELION

"It was strong and beautiful, with wide-spreading branches, for its roots went deep into abundant water." —Ezekiel 31:7(NLT)

We have roots in our lives that are good, and we have roots that are not so good. The root represents the cause, the foundation, or the life source of every circumstance. It is the lifeline of what is actually seen. In order to alleviate what is seen we need to destroy and replace some of the roots in our lives; just like with the dandelions in our yards.

The dandelion is a tough weed. This is a flower that once it seeds, if left alone, will eventually consume the yard. When we make a decision on how to destroy the dandelion, if we don't understand its nature, the only thing we can resort to is our own common sense, which says mow the lawn or cut the flower. But the problem is that this is only a temporary solution. What we are really doing when we cut the flower is dealing with what can be seen on the surface. And what can be seen is only evidence that there is something deeper. The flower is connected to the root system of the plant, and until the root is destroyed the flower will keep coming back. Once the root is destroyed the flower simply dies.

When it comes to losing excess body fat many of us resort to the latest fad diet. We deal with what can be seen, which is the excess body fat. So we do what we have been taught, which is to cut calories and exercise, but this is only a surface solution. The excess fat is what can be seen (or the surface) and is only evidence that there is something deeper. In order to be successful, we must do exactly what is done with the dandelion, which is going to the root and destroying it.

By not dealing with the root of the problem all of our dieting efforts usually end in failure. If we continue to deal with the symptom, which is the excess body fat, it will keep coming back. Each time we lose body fat without discovering the root and destroying it our metabolism suffers. This makes fat loss that much more difficult the next time.

Dandelions and excess body fat have the following similarities:
- If the root is not destroyed both the dandelion and the body fat will return.
- Each time we deal with what we see (the flower or the excess body fat), and not "the root," when it comes back it's tougher and harder to destroy.
- If not effectively addressed they will increase in size and number.
- In order to overcome excess body fat, and the dandelion, you must have appropriate knowledge.
- Dealing with the surface brings a short-term sense of security because you will think the problem is gone when it's actually still there and will soon resurface.

In order to develop an effective solution for any problem we must first discover its origin or "the root." Throughout this section of the book we are going to unveil many root causes of excess body fat.

Each individual has different circumstances in their lives, which present different challenges, and if you are carrying excess body fat there are most likely multiple root causes. This section will help you discover the root or roots and aid you in finding an effective solution that will help you to achieve permanent fat loss.

In the following chapter, you will learn that the root causes of excess body fat are stumbling blocks that, unless removed, will prevent you from reaching your ultimate goals.

Chapter 3

STUMBLING BLOCKS

"Cast ye up, cast ye up, prepare the way, take up the stumbling block(s) out of the way of my people." —Isaiah 57: 14

Stumbling Blocks ("Roots") are issues or circumstances that obstruct, or become obstacles, with the intention of crippling and preventing you from reaching your goals. A stumbling block can also be a diversion to distract you from God's truth concerning your life; an interference to reaching your God-given potential. Stumbling blocks are the main cause of our fat-loss problems.

There are two types of stumbling blocks that can prevent you from permanently losing body fat. The first is a hindrance, which is a physical or natural stumbling block. The second is a spiritual or emotional stumbling block. I refer to this as a soul wound.

Hindrances – Hindrances are natural or physical stumbling blocks that primarily come from outside sources penetrating the mind or the intellect. They affect you mentally and physically. This type of stumbling block can be dealt with and dispelled intellectually.

You overcome a hindrance by understanding your old counter-productive thought process and replacing it with accurate knowledge, so that you can send your body the appropriate fat loss signals. After you embrace and apply true science, concerning the matter, you will achieve results.

Soul Wounds – Soul wounds are spiritual stumbling blocks that also come from outside sources. But they penetrate deeper, not only affecting the mind, but they create wounds to the heart and soul. They affect you mentally, emotionally, spiritually, and physically. Soul wounds are more difficult to rectify because the stumbling block is caused by an injury deep within. They must be ministered to spiritually by acknowledging and releasing the root of the hurt, coupled with prayer for God's deliverance. The Lord is the only one capable of healing a wound to the soul.

HINDRANCE OR SOUL WOUND?

Throughout our lives there are many situations in which hindrances or soul wounds can occur. Sometimes we are unable to determine whether a particular stumbling block is a hindrance or a soul wound. A hindrance and a soul wound may be interwoven because a soul wound is often inflicted through the doorway of the mind. Remember, a hindrance is easily dealt with because all we need is a change of mind or a new thought process, but a soul wound requires much more than a change of thought. The key to identifying the type of stumbling block you are dealing with is by discovering its root.

Depression is one example of a stumbling block that can be either a hindrance or a soul wound. If your depression originates from a mental source, such as being overwhelmed with daily tasks, it is a hindrance. If your depression originates from an emotional source, like an abusive relationship, it is a soul wound.

You must establish whether you are dealing with a hindrance or a soul wound, so you can know how to effectively address the problem. If a soul wound is dealt with like a hindrance, it is like putting a Band-Aid over a malignant cancer — the band-aid is not equipped to heal cancer.

A stumbling block resulting from misinformation can be resolved by acquiring appropriate knowledge. With a soul wound, all the knowledge in the world cannot heal the problem. Only God can.

We want to bring this into perspective and provide you with a visual that makes this concept easy to understand. Let's paint a picture of two individuals starting at the same place in which both of them desire to decrease body fat, but one has a struggle with a hindrance and the other suffers with a soul wound:

Lucy is protected by parents, family, and friends; but has struggled with yo-yo dieting for twenty-five years due to misinformation about nutrition. She has been hindered from achieving effective permanent fat loss.

Deborah is completely unprotected: emotionally, physically, and spiritually. She encountered several abuses during the previous twenty-five years of her life. She was raped as a child, and neglected by her parents. Because of her previous abuse, she attracted abusive boyfriends. She put on excess body fat as a sub-conscious protective mechanism.

Lucy's struggle with obesity is a hindrance that can be turned around simply by acquiring appropriate knowledge and praying for discipline. Deborah, on the other hand, suffers from a deep soul wound. No amount of knowledge about nutrition will help Deborah permanently lose excess body fat. Deborah needs spiritual attention.

Lay Aside Every Weight

One mistake many of us make is we try to separate the physical from the spiritual, not realizing the connection. Whatever affects you mentally, emotionally, and spiritually will affect you physically. By the same token, what affects you physically will also affect you mentally, emotionally, and spiritually. These stumbling blocks, whether they are hindrances or soul wounds, can create excess weight physically and spiritually. The Bible says in Hebrews 12:1, *"Let us lay aside every weight, and the sin which doth so easily beset us, and let us run with patience the race that is set before us."* God's desire is for us to lay aside every "weight and sin" that hinders us. The adversary's desire, on the other hand, is for us to accumulate as much excess weight as possible, physically and spiritually, because he understands that this will hold us back on every level. God wants us to have a life of balance. Stability and balance may seem hard to find, but with God's help we can do what seems impossible {Proverbs 11:1; 20:23}.

Man's opinions and misinformation have created massive confusion that only compounds the problem of being unhealthy, overweight, or obese. In order to dispel the confusion, you must gain an understanding of how fat loss works by learning the facts concerning the stumbling blocks that have caused you to become overweight or obese. In Hosea 4:6 God says, *"My people perish for lack of knowledge."* God is not saying, "My people perish for lack of information." The problem is we have way too much information, but a great deal of it has been incorrect and void of God's power. When God speaks of knowledge in Hosea, He is referring to knowledge concerning Him and His Word. When God's Word is involved, God Himself supplies the power to fulfill what He says. He says, *"My Word is settled in Heaven,"* so Heaven has already made a stance on earthly circumstances. If you are struggling with losing excess body fat, you need to agree with God's stance concerning your health and fat loss and trust Him to bring it to pass – this is the only solution to permanent fat loss and true transformation.

The next four chapters will help you identify your personal stumbling blocks, so you can effectively apply the appropriate solution to overcoming your struggle with excess body fat. Understanding the "root" of your struggle is not an excuse to continue being overweight or obese. It provides an explanation for why you have been unsuccessful in your attempts to achieve permanent fat loss. Once you identify the underlying reason, you will be better equipped to plan the correct strategy and win the battle.

But first, I would like to pray for your success:

Lord, I thank You for their deliverance. I thank You for their success. I thank You for giving them appropriate knowledge and understanding. Confusion must be dispelled in order for them to be effective in their quest for successful fat loss, physically and spiritually. I ask You to reveal every hindrance that would stop them from being effective. I ask You to reveal every soul wound that has afflicted them. Heal their secret pain; dry the eyes that cry lonely tears over soul wounds that penetrate deeply. Give them the humility that is necessary so that You might heal them. Release them from any pride that may cause them to be distant from You. Thank You for helping them to understand that their struggle with being overweight has a deeper root cause. Help them to realize that it's not a lack of willpower that keeps them from success. We all need Your power. I thank You in advance for their victory. In Jesus' name. Amen.

There are many stumbling blocks related to being overweight or obese. Just as stated before you must determine the root cause. Let God help you identify, face, and stand up to the hindrances and soul wounds that caused you to put on the excess body fat. Then, once and for all, you can overcome the stumbling blocks that have kept you from successfully decreasing body fat.

Chapter 4

HINDRANCES

"Who did hinder you that you did not obey the truth?
—Galatians 5:7

There is no need for you to be hindered in your pursuit to decrease body fat because God has provided accurate knowledge for us concerning diet and nutrition, exercise, health, and longevity. The question in Galatians is, *"Who did hinder you that you did not obey the truth,"* meaning God's Word. We have been hindered by following man's methods, schemes, and devices concerning our desire to effectively decrease excess body fat. The Bible tells us to acknowledge God in <u>all</u> of our ways and He will direct our path {Proverbs 3:6}.

Man's limited knowledge and inaccurate attempts for long term fat loss and health are left wanting when compared to God's truth, which is found in Scripture. We are inundated with information that can lead to confusion. All we need is God's accurate and effective knowledge, which will bring success in our quest for permanent fat loss.

Remember, hindrances are natural or physical stumbling blocks that primarily come from an outside source that penetrate the mind or the intellect. They affect you mentally and physically. The important thing about a hindrance is that it can be rectified by acquiring accurate knowledge and prayer.

When it comes to being overweight or obese many people fail to recognize the health risks. The main concern is how they look and how others see them. Out of desperation, it is easy to gravitate toward diets that promote quick and easy fat loss by using unhealthy gimmicks. Taking the approach of attacking what you see, creates a bigger problem that will be harder to deal with in the future. Though you may experience temporary weight loss, you are statistically guaranteed to put the weight you have lost back on, plus a few more pounds.

You will never be successful with permanent fat loss until you pinpoint and deal with the root of the problem. I have identified seven categories of hindrances that are most commonly found in those struggling with excess body fat:

- ❑ Lack of Appropriate Knowledge
- ❑ Self-help
- ❑ Modern Lifestyles and Behaviors
- ❑ Fad Dieting
- ❑ Toxic Foods
- ❑ Discouragement
- ❑ The Hormone Hindrance: For Men & Women

HINDRANCE #1: LACK OF APPROPRIATE KNOWLEDGE

A maze of information enters our homes every day through television, the Internet, magazines, diet and nutrition books, fitness and fat-loss programs, and nutrition experts. We may notice one expert has the opinion that decreasing fat in our diet will cause us to decrease body fat. This opinion is stated as fact in books, in articles, and on TV programs. Another expert tells us that a decrease in carbohydrates is the key to fat loss; this too is stated in the media as being factual.

Consumers become rightfully confused. We ask ourselves after trying both solutions – unsuccessfully – "Who or what can I believe, since previous experts have proven themselves to be wrong?" Just because something is in print, does not make it a fact. Just because an expert or a celebrity makes a convincing statement, does not make it a fact. We tend to believe it is a fact because the source seems to be credible, they appear to be knowledgeable, and they are definitely convincing.

You, as the consumer, have the responsibility to find out if you are dealing with an opinion that has an emotional draw, a well-meaning zealous individual touting inaccurate information, or a true fact. With that said, let's look at what a fact really is. A fact is information that is infallible or perfect. A fact is something that is concrete and can't be changed. A fact is the truth; Jesus said, "*I am the truth.*" Do you want to follow man's opinions, which may be stated as a fact; or God's truth, which is perfect, infallible, without error or room to be changed?

Hindrance #2: Self-Help

If you think about it, self-help is a ridiculous concept. *Self* means you all alone. *Help* is a cry for assistance from something outside of oneself. Stop for a moment and think about the definition of these two words – they are opposite. Self-help, by the nature of the word, is an outward admission that help is needed. It is a good thing to acknowledge that you need help; it is unreasonable to expect to find the help you need within yourself.

When we acknowledge that help is needed, we are doing what we were created to do according to God's design. Hebrews 13:6 says, "*So that we may boldly say, the Lord is my helper.*"

Many people are searching for help through other resource rather than God, such as self-help books, seminars, music, holistic healings, and psychic readings. These resources instruct people to look within to find help. If you are honest with yourself, regardless of how many times you revisit the seminars, tapes, books, and teachings, you find yourself in the same situation – in need of help. The reason you revisit these tools of self-help is because in the beginning these things may give you an emotional high, but they have no sustaining impact to influence a permanent change. If all you have to depend on is the limited ability you have within yourself, you will always be disappointed and discouraged.

There are times when you may feel helpless and hopeless. At these times you can turn to the Lord because He wants to help you. The Bible says that all things are possible to those who believe. God is the only source of power that has no limitations, knows no failure, and is able to meet all of your needs.

Nothing can be effectively done, directly or indirectly, without Him. In John 15:5 the Lord says, *"Without me you can do <u>nothing</u>."* The answer to our problems is not self-help, but God's help.

HINDRANCE #3: MODERN LIFESTYLES AND BEHAVIORS

If we could travel back in time just a few decades, we would be amazed at the difference in the waist sizes of the population. Thirty years ago, very few people were morbidly obese, but today this has become commonplace. Morbid obesity is defined as having a Body Mass Index (BMI) of 40 percent or above, or one hundred pounds over a healthy body weight.

Being overweight and obese has become a worldwide epidemic in the past thirty years. Many people are convinced that being overweight or obese is their fate, claiming it is a genetic disposition. With this being said, consider that most of the adults who are alive today were also alive thirty years ago, when obesity rates were dramatically lower. During the last three decades our genetic make-up hasn't changed, but our lifestyles and behaviors have. Environment, developed habits, and behaviors have strongly influenced the increase of obesity.

Due to modern technology we have become more inactive in work and play. Many jobs require more brainpower and less manpower. A large part of our population sits behind a desk working with computers and cell phones, using elevators and escalators. Even our labor-intensive jobs are much less physically challenging. We no longer have to dig with a shovel; we have machines that can dig a hole faster and more efficiently. We no longer need a hammer to drive nails; we have nail guns to do the job for us. The modern high-tech environment we have created in the workplace is conducive to making us overweight and obese.

Our play and recreation time has also been affected by our high-tech, fast-paced society. Take golf, for instance. At one time golf was considered good for cardiovascular and resistance training. Then the golf cart replaced walking and carrying a thirty-to-forty-pound golf bag for eighteen holes.

Significant tradeoffs have been made in our recreational activities. Many of these activities increase the exercise of the mind, but decrease physical activity. Surfing the Net, chatting online, watching TV, and playing video games have taken the place of hide-and-go-seek, jumping rope, and other childhood activities that increase metabolism and burn fat.

Our children used to play on scooters that required standing and using their own strength and energy to operate. Today we have scooters that have chairs to sit on and motors that deprive the child from using his own energy. When the child uses his own energy, it is called exercise, this helps to increase his metabolism and enhances his health. As we can plainly see, the advancement of technology has greatly affected all areas of our lives. In becoming a high tech society, our sacrifice has been much too great.

Overall, we are at the highest point in history for being overweight and obese; at the same time, we are at the lowest point for physical activity and good health. We are simply not getting enough physical activity and exercise.

In today's busy world, it is easy to justify not exercising. The mere thought of adding one more thing into our lives can be mentally exhausting. The common excuse is that there are not enough hours in the day. Therefore, we commit to our personal responsibilities and to satisfying the immediate needs of others. By not classifying exercise as one of our primary needs we are neglecting our health and contributing to the increase of body fat. If you neglect your health, the people you want to take care of will end up with the obligation of taking care of you.

If you think becoming healthy and fit requires an enormous amount of time, be encouraged that your thought process is simply wrong. The key to becoming healthy and fit is to have a consistent exercise program that fits into your busy life, without neglecting your other obligations.

The hindrance of our modern lifestyles and behaviors can easily be overcome, but it requires more than just good time management and will-power. It can be difficult to prioritize what's most important. Through prayer, allow God to be involved with your decisions. He will help you create balance between fulfilling your responsibilities and taking care of those you love.

HINDRANCE #4: FAD DIETING

Fad dieting is a food regimen designed for weight loss that is widely accepted by society. Yet most fad diets are unhealthy, depriving the body of nutrients necessary for health and longevity. A common pattern of these diets is that they leave out entire food groups.

Other fad diets cut calories so low that you are deprived of energy. In order to compensate for the lack of calories your body will convert muscle protein into sugar to be used as energy. The body will adjust over time and when it finally regulates itself to the decrease in calories, you can be sure your metabolism has been considerably damaged. Fad dieting causes the metabolism to become sluggish, resulting in fat gain. When you begin to decrease or fluctuate caloric intake, your body goes into a self-preservation state. The number one objective for the body is survival. When you change your eating habits (such as, increasing protein, decreasing fat, cutting carbohydrates, etc.) the body will adapt to the new food regimen and resort to a survival mode.

Fad dieting might result in temporary weight loss, but the long-term result is fat gain. The following is a brief list of yo-yo fad diets that have proven to be ineffective:

- ❑ Low-carbohydrate/high-protein diets
- ❑ Low-fat diets
- ❑ Cabbage Soup Diet
- ❑ Cider vinegar diet
- ❑ Crash diets
- ❑ The Hollywood Forty-Eight-Hour Diet

HINDRANCE #5: TOXIC FOODS

Most of today's grocery stores and fast-food restaurants have become a major hindrance in our ability to achieve and maintain healthy, fit, and lean bodies. Often, convenience takes priority. The problem with convenient meals is that you end up eating large amounts of food that are high in calories and fat; and taste and convenience are placed ahead of the nutri-tion needed for reaching your health and fat loss goals. The condition of our health and physical bodies is evidence that many people are malnour-ished and mis-nourished. This is caused by consuming high-calorie diets that are deficient in essential vitamins and nutrients.

It is easy to make poor nutritional choices if you don't have a plan in place. Over time, poor choices turn into bad eating habits and increased waist sizes. If you're not committed to a specific eating plan that has be-come a permanent lifestyle, you will be enticed with tempting foods that are filled with toxins by friends, family, and fellow employees who are simply making a kind gesture, not realizing how detrimental it is to your health and fat loss goals.

In order to overcome the hindrances attached to food, we must exam-ine the ones that negatively affect our health and cause an increase of body fat, then make a decision to avoid those choices.

Food Cravings and Addictions

One of the major downfalls in our quest to decrease body fat is fighting off undesired food cravings and addictions. Before we can get a complete understanding of the effects of cravings and addictions, it is important to understand what they are and where they come from. A food craving is an insatiable desire for something edible. Cravings are derived from physical, mental, and emotional sources. A physical food craving may be caused by a hormonal imbalance in the body, such as a lack of serotonin, dopamine, or leptin. A mental food craving can be created in the subconscious mind, such as a bad habit. An emotional food craving is developed through a negative experience, such as a broken heart. The difference between a crav-ing and a food addiction is that a food addiction is associated with a depen-dence that has absolutely nothing to do with will-power. A high percentage of the population suffers with food addictions and don't realize it. If you are not sure, but want to determine if you are addicted to food, ask yourself this simple question. If you miss a meal or two, does it result in headaches, irritability, nervousness, low energy, depression, or nausea? If so, you may be struggling with a food addiction. If food cravings or addictions exist in your life, and are not brought under control, this situation alone could cause you to become overweight or obese.

Some of the things that cause cravings and addictions are highly refined sugars, sugar substitutes, and MSG, which are prevalent in today's processed foods and fast foods.

High-Fructose Corn Syrup

High-Fructose Corn Syrup (HFCS) is a natural sugar that has been fractionated, chemically processed, and concentrated. This process causes it to become very fattening and dangerous to our health. It is one of the most addictive substances in our diet today.

The consumption of HFCS has increased dramatically in the last twenty-five years (hand-in-hand with the obesity epidemic) and has infiltrated the entire food industry. It is found in a large percentage of the foods on our grocery store shelves.

One reason HFCS is so widely used is that it tastes much sweeter than sugar; therefore, less is required to adequately sweeten products. It is also much less expensive to produce, and the government subsidizes the farming of corn, further lowering the cost. HFCS is also a preservative that extends shelf life. But high-fructose corn syrup is known to contribute to insulin resistance, increased calorie intake, impaired metabolism, weight gain, high cholesterol, and high blood pressure. We may not be able to completely avoid this product, but it is important we are aware of its effects so we can limit our consumption.

Sugar Substitutes

Sugar substitutes (such as aspartame, sucralose, and saccharin) are even worse for your health than HFCS and are very deceptive. They have been touted to yield no calories, causing the average person to believe that products containing these substances will help them in their desire to decrease body fat. The problem with this theory is that the body's digestive enzymes are only designed to absorb and digest the three macronutrients: proteins, fats, and carbohydrates. When something sweet comes into the mouth, a signal is sent to the brain that a simple carbohydrate has entered the body; therefore, digestion begins. The problem is the sugar substitutes have no calories to digest, so this disrupts the body's chemistry. The false signal that was sent to the brain causes an increase in appetite and cravings. Not only do these artificial sweeteners lack the ability to assist in decreasing body fat, but they are also known to be detrimental to our health.

Soft Drinks

Soft drinks have widely contributed to the epidemic of being overweight and obese. According to the National Soft Drink Association, consumption of soft drinks is now over six hundred twelve-ounce servings per person per year.

Soft drinks are sweetened by some of the most dangerous sweeteners; such as, high-fructose corn syrup or sugar substitutes. When sugar or sugar substitutes are ingested in liquid form they enter the bloodstream more rapidly than in a solid.

In 1984, the major soft-drink corporations switched to HFCS from the more expensive, safe, natural sugars. Since then there has been a dramatic increase in the consumption of soft drinks. Some of the health risks associated with the consumption of soft drinks are diabetes, high cholesterol, osteoporosis, bone fractures, nutritional deficiencies, heart disease, food addictions, neurotransmitter dysfunction from the chemical sweeteners, life-changing hormonal disturbances, and being overweight and obese. If you are trying to increase your health and decrease body fat, **avoid soft drinks completely.**

Fast-Food and Groceries

We have addressed some specific hindrances pertaining to food, but this would not be complete without including fast food and our local grocery stores. Over the past thirty-six years, we have made a major shift from healthy home-cooked meals to convenient, fattening, high-calorie, super-sized-portion fast foods. Our busy, fast-paced lifestyles limit the time we have available for healthy food preparation. The fast-food industry has accommodated this demand by providing foods that are prepared with speed and uniformity.

Fast food, by the nature of the word, means to be eaten "on the go." Fast foods are often full of ingredients designed for taste, consistency, and freshness. Although fast foods are convenient for our hectic lifestyles, they come with a high price, which is being overweight and obese, and having an increased risk of cancer and other health ailments.

One of the main causes of excess body fat is eating nutrient-deficient, high-calorie meals loaded with high-fructose corn syrup, hydrogenated vegetables oils, and MSG. These ingredients are found in most fast food selections. Conventional restaurants also use these fattening, highly addictive substances.

Our neighborhood grocery stores also contribute to our becoming overweight and obese. At one time, grocery shelves were filled with foods that were safe and nourishing. Today we are bombarded with false advertisements, deceptive schemes, and labels designed to gain our hard-earned dollars. We must read labels and examine the content. Here are a few ingredients that should be avoided:

- ❑ Enriched flours
- ❑ High-fructose corn syrup
- ❑ Partially hydrogenated soybean oil
- ❑ Homogenized dairy products
- ❑ Sugar substitutes (Ex., Aspartame, Sucralose, and Saccharin)
- ❑ MSG

The average person already has a career and has no desire to become a well versed food scientist, nutritionist, or someone who is proficient in reading labels and understanding ingredients. The problem is our foods are allowed to be sold in an unhealthy state. We need a dependable organization that will stand up and monitor what is allowed to be sold on the grocery store shelves. Until that takes place we need to take the initiative to protect ourselves and our families.

HINDRANCE #6: DISCOURAGEMENT

When each new fat-loss diet comes along, we try it, hoping this will finally be the solution to permanent fat loss. Each time, our failure brings about a deeper discouragement, which makes it harder to muster up the courage to try again.

If you are discouraged by your previous failed attempts to attain permanent fat loss, you are not alone. Almost every adult in this country has been on diets that haven't worked, taken weight-loss pills that were a waste of money, and bought exercise equipment they didn't use consistently. Some have even been convinced to try self-help techniques; such as positive thinking and using pure willpower to make their excess body fat simply melt away. Yet the weight continues to increase and your body continues to expand.

Of course you're discouraged. Who wouldn't be? You need to know that all of your failed attempts have no jurisdiction over your future success. It is ok for you to admit that you have failed in the past, but this does not label you as a failure. The only time you can't afford to fail is the last time you try.

To be successful in the area of fat loss, you just need to find the right formula and allow God to help you implement it. If you follow God's successful formula for physical and spiritual fat loss through a life transformation, there will be no need to try again!

We pray that this chapter has been a real eye opener and revealed some of the hindrances that you have faced in your past attempts to achieve permanent fat loss. **The final hindrance has affected the majority of the population in one way or another and is called — The Hormone Hindrance (For Men and Women).** It has the ability to completely disrupt lives and cause obesity single-handedly. This final hindrance is so complex that I have devoted the entire next chapter to it.

Chapter 5

THE HORMONE HINDRANCE

for Men & Women

If you are overweight or obese, an overstressed endocrine system may be the root cause. At least 80 percent of individuals who are overweight or obese struggle with losing excess body fat partially because of endocrine-related issues. If you are one of those numbered in this statistic you will be glad to know endocrine and hormone related obesity can be reversed.

The endocrine system is vital in fat metabolism and losing excess body fat. If certain factors exist within the endocrine system it literally becomes impossible for you to decrease body fat long-term. All the diets in the world won't make much of a difference in achieving healthy, lasting results.

The human body needs more than fifty hormones to function properly. These hormones are produced and secreted by the endocrine system. This delicate system influences every function of the body, including heartbeat, eye movement, cell growth (both fat and muscle), emotions, learning ability, and metabolism. This vital system can become over-stressed due to mental exhaustion, physical burn-out, vitamin and mineral deficiency, and the toxic chemicals found in many foods. The counter-productive secretion (either too much or too little) of certain hormones can affect excess body fat. <u>These fat-causing hormone secretions are affected by what you eat, how much you eat, the times you eat, the combinations of what you eat, your activities, and the stress in your life.</u>

Five major endocrine glands secrete hormones that contribute to the increase or decrease of body fat. Without the proper nutrients our bodies cannot produce these essential life giving hormones. In this section, I will explain the function of each of these glands and how they are affected by nutrition, as well as lack of nutrition. This will give you an appreciation and understanding of how important and delicate the endocrine system really is, and your need to safeguard it. In the illustration, the five major glands are shown.

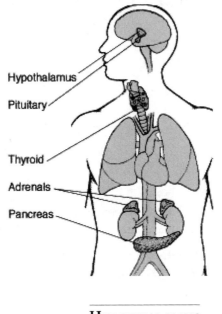

HYPOTHALAMUS

The hypothalamus is located in the brain. It is one of the most delicate of all the hormone-secreting glands in the endocrine system. Even though the hypothalamus is a very small gland (about the size of an almond), it is responsible for many vital functions of the body, including the control of hunger, thirst, and satiety. And it regulates various activities in the body connected with metabolism. The hypothalamus also assists the actions of the pituitary gland.

This small gland performed its functions just fine when people ate the foods originally created by God. Today the hypothalamus is exposed to excitotoxins; such as monosodium glutamate (MSG) and aspartame. These toxins are found in many of the foods we eat. These chemicals have the ability to completely alter the body's chemistry and cause significant damage to our health, in addition to accelerating body fat. One way these chemicals affect the endocrine system is by creating lesions on the hypo-thalamus. Once the hypothalamus is damaged from exposure to MSG, aspartame, and other excitotoxins, it no longer sends or receives signals properly.

One of the functions of the hypothalamus is to send a signal to the brain that the body is full, but if it is damaged it loses its ability to medi-ate between the body and the brain. Leptin is a hormone that transmits a signal to the hypothalamus that the body is full. The hypothalamus then relays that signal to the brain. If your hypothalamus is injured, from the lesions caused by the toxic chemicals, the leptin signal will be ignored. Thus you will continue to crave more calories, never feeling satisfied. Even though the body has received adequate amounts of food, you feel a sense of urgency to eat — as if you hadn't eaten at all.

We can't leave it to chance that the food industry is looking out for our health. It is important for us to have accurate knowledge so we can make educated, healthy decisions concerning the substances we put in our mouth and the way we feed our families. The following is a recommended regimen to reverse damage to the hypothalamus:

- Check food labels in order to avoid MSG and aspartame. (See Exhibit 1 in the back of the book for a comprehensive list of dis-guised names for MSG.)
- Get six to eight hours of sleep per night, so the body can experi-ence delta sleep, which is mandatory for adequate recovery and natural healing.
- Eat well-balanced meals containing foods that are as close to their original state as possible to rejuvenate, build, and promote health and longevity.
- Take supplements that promote healing of the hypothalamus. (For more information, see the chapter on supplementation.)

Supplement Recommendations are:
- Phosphotydil Serine: A very effective protector against glutamate (MSG) toxicity.

- Vitamin C: A major player in protecting the brain from free radical damage.
- Selenium: An antioxidant which contributes to healing of the hypothalamus.
- Eleutherococcus Senticosus: Eleuthero is useful when the hypothalamus is depleted. Symptoms of this condition include fatigue, stress, neurasthenia, and sore muscles associated with the hypofunctioning of the endocrine system. Eleutherococcus may alleviate these symptoms. {Wikipedia.org}

PITUITARY GLAND

The endocrine system is like an orchestra, the conductor being the pea-sized gland called the pituitary gland. It is often referred to as the master gland because it controls the functions of most other endocrine glands. The pituitary gland is found at the base of the brain, beneath the hypothalamus.

The hormones secreted from the pituitary gland help control many bodily processes, including growth, water regulation, blood pressure, sex organ function, and metabolism. The pituitary signals the thyroid and the adrenal glands to secrete the necessary hormones for optimal bodily function, and it indirectly signals the pancreas through the liver.

If the pituitary is damaged through a bombardment of high-fructose corn syrup, excitotoxins (such as, MSG and Aspartame), and other damaging chemicals; the entire endocrine system is compromised and begins to malfunction. This creates a domino effect, causing mental, emotional, and physical problems, including an increase in unwanted body fat.

A healthy pituitary gland releases growth hormone that increases muscle mass and bone density. Once damage occurs to the pituitary, this growth hormone is diminished, resulting in decreased muscle mass and increased body fat.

You can limit the amount of excitotoxins and dangerous chemicals you ingest by reading the labels on the foods you buy. **Note**: It is impossible to completely avoid these dangerous substances because they are so widespread and are disguised with tricky names.

With this being said, it is absolutely necessary to supplement your food with good nutritional whole food supplementation and sufficient amounts of high-quality vitamins and minerals. This will assist in warding off the negative effects of excitotoxins, reversing nutritional deficiencies, and decreasing exhaustion of the pituitary gland.

There are three avenues to effectively increase the release of natural growth hormone from the pituitary. These are:

- Strenuous anaerobic exercise (especially heavy squats, heavy dead lifts, and sprints)
- Delta sleep (this is the first hour of deep sleep)
- L-Triptaphane, L-Ornithine, and L-Arginine (these are amino acids that can be supplemented to assist in releasing human growth hormone naturally. They must be ingested individually, without the presence of the other amino acids)

THYROID

The thyroid is a butterfly-shaped gland located in the front part of the lower neck. The thyroid is considered to be the body's thermostat. It is responsible for secreting hormones that regulate body temperature. Body temperature (or metabolism) directly relates to how much energy is being used. A high metabolism creates an inferno-like effect that demands the body to burn more calories, thus requiring more protein, fats, and carbohydrates to sustain itself. On the other hand, a body with a low metabolism requires fewer calories. It is common for someone with a low metabolism to put on a considerable amount of excess body fat in a short period of time while eating a normal diet. This is another major contributor to the overweight and obesity epidemic.

The condition of a low metabolism is called hypothyroidism. Some of the characteristics of this disease are low energy, unwarranted depression, cold intolerance, and excessive weight gain.

Many overweight and obese people have low iodine utilization and hypothyroidism. A high percentage of the adult population that carries excess body fat is affected by at least one of these conditions.

A low thyroid is caused by thyroid exhaustion, iodine deficiency, toxic chemicals in our food and water, and excessive amounts of estrogen. Following is a brief explanation of the main contributors to hypothyroidism, and the solutions you can implement to reverse it.

Thyroid Exhaustion

Thyroid exhaustion is caused by extreme fatigue due to lack of sleep, overexposure to severe weather conditions, and the emotional, mental, and physical stress that comes from everyday life. To heal the thyroid from exhaustion, you must get proper rest, which will probably require the practice of effective time-management techniques. Oftentimes, stressful circumstances cannot be avoided, but you can always improve the way you deal with them. Know your limitations in stressful circumstances, do what you can to resolve them, and turn the rest over to God in prayer.

Iodine Deficiency

Iodine is required to produce thyroid hormones. It is also required in the fat cell, so they have the ability to reduce in size. If your body is iodine deficient, it has a tendency to rapidly accumulate excess body fat. If you eat a normal diet and do not have proper levels of iodine these low levels increase your probability of carrying excess body fat.

The average American ingests approximately 150 mcg. of iodine daily, which is insufficient for optimal thyroid function. Safe, effective, and natural alternatives for assisting in the reversal of iodine deficiencies and healing the thyroid gland; include high doses of iodine for a short period of time, high doses of vitamin C, eating unrefined sea salt, taking Epsom salt baths, and ionic mineral supplementation.

Toxic Chemicals

The toxic chemicals we are referring to are the halogens – fluorine, chlorine, perchlorate, and bromine. These toxic substances are bioaccumulative, which means they build up in the body, mainly in the fat cells.

These halogens bind to the iodine receptors of the fat cell and block the function of the thyroid hormones. What this means to you is when a cell is filled with iodine, it has the natural ability to decrease fat. If the cell is filled with halogens fat reduction is difficult, if not impossible, to achieve, even on a diet and exercise program. The body actually becomes fat loss resistant.

These halogens can be found in a wide variety of places. For example, healthy iodine was once a common ingredient in breads and baked goods. Today it has been exchanged for unhealthy bromine, which is a poison and has no place in human consumption. These destructive halogens can also be found in processed white flour, drinking water, swimming pools, some sports and soft drinks, salt, artificial sweeteners, cow's milk, toothpaste, and prescription medications.

There are several things you can do to control the amount of dangerous halogens consumed, or that have accumulated in your body:

1. Read labels and steer away from products with halogens.
2. Complete the Faith & Fat Loss Twenty-One Day Detoxification Program to rid the body of the accumulated toxins.
3. Take a high-quality source of natural iodine. (See the chapter on supplementation)

Estrogen Dominance

Estrogen dominance takes place when an excessive amount of estrogen is present in the body. Estrogen is a necessary hormone and is naturally secreted in higher amounts in women than in men. Estrogen is necessary for childbearing and causes feminine attributes, such as breast tissue growth and a curvy body. An excessive amount of estrogen can override the natural signals of other hormones and increase body fat as well as causing feminine attributes.

High levels of estrogen come from a combination of the following three primary sources:

1. Naturally occurring estrogen that is produced in the body by the endocrine system
2. Phytoestrogens (*phyto* means plant) are naturally occurring and imitate estrogen functions in the body (found in a variety of plants, herbs, and spices)
3. Xenoestrogens (*xeno* means foreign) are man-made toxic chemicals that mimic estrogen in the body and are produced by the thousands (these toxins are found in many foods, water, medications, cleaning supplies, plastics, cosmetics, and toiletries)

In our society today, men and women have an overabundance of estrogen that is so far out of balance, the body can't handle it. This causes a wide variety of health, obesity, and gender-altering issues.

Below are some of the effects of estrogen dominance:

In Women

Excess estrogen causes hormonal imbalances that contribute to emotional problems, depression, bipolar disorder, etc. It also causes water retention, fatigue, loss of vigor, and **tremendous fat gain. The type of fat gained from excessive amounts of estrogen resists weight loss**.

Estrogen dominance can interfere with thyroid hormone activity and is often a primary underlying cause of thyroid dysfunction. Estrogen and thyroid hormones oppose each other. Estrogen is designed to maintain and increase body fat; whereas thyroid hormones are designed to increase metabolism, causing a decrease in body fat. Excess estrogen will prevent the thyroid from doing its job and can result in hypothyroid symptoms, including the rapid increase of excess body fat.

In Men

When a man is plagued with an overabundance of estrogen it begins to dominate his body, creating female attributes. Increased estrogen levels can cause reduced sperm count, hair loss, impotency, and the growth of female breast tissue.

The growth of female breast tissue is called, *Gynecomastia*. Although it is rarely talked about, it affects 40 to 60 percent of men in the United States. Once breast tissue has developed it's very difficult to eliminate. Breast reduction surgery is one of the most prevalent cosmetic surgeries for men. This condition also has a profound effect on teenage boys. In the US, fourteen thousand young men have breast reduction surgery each year.

Previously, we covered the necessity of estrogen that naturally occurs in the body, which is produced by the endocrine system. We also discussed the danger of the over-abundance of estrogen that is derived from the combination of the phytoestrogens and the xenoestrogens (known as estrogen mimickers). If we were to eliminate any one of these sources of estrogen, the threat of estrogen dominance would be reduced. The problem lies in the "cocktail effect," meaning the multiple sources that are introduced into the body on a daily basis. Below is a short list of the estrogens found in our environment that overwhelm the body:

<u>**Phytoestrogens:**</u> (an inferior natural form of estrogen)

- Soy products (soy milk, tofu, vegetable protein, etc.)
- Flaxseeds
- Vegetable oils (safflower oil, canola oil, margarine, etc.)
- Red clover
- Black cohosh
- Chasteberry
- Dong quai

Xenoestrogens: (A bioaccumulative dangerous toxic chemical that mimicks estrogen)

- Commercially raised meats (hormone-and-antibiotic injected)
- Hormone-and-antibiotic injected dairy products
- Canned and processed foods
- Petroleum-based products
- Plastic containers and plastic food wrap
- Personal-care products
- Insecticides, pesticides, herbicides, fungicides
- Chemical cleaners
- Tap water

Correcting Estrogen Dominance

To avoid or correct estrogen dominance, follow these guidelines:

- Eat vegetables that are high in fiber.
- Drink distilled water fortified with ionic minerals to eliminate the pesticides.
- Eat organic fruits and vegetables, when possible, or thoroughly wash your fruits and vegetables before eating.
- Eat cruciferous vegetables that are slightly steamed. (This releases the active estrogen-inhibiting enzymes.)
- Eat citrus fruits.
- Eat grass-fed or hormone-free meats. (If you purchase meat from another source, trim off the fat – estrogen mimickers accumulate in the fat.)
- Avoid processed meats.
- Eat eggs from cage free chickens.
- Eat broccoli, cabbage, brussels sprouts, radishes, onions, and garlic.
- Drink chamomile tea.
- Do not microwave foods in plastic containers or cover with plastic wrap.

- Do not drink water that is bottled in plastic that has been exposed to heat; such as, being left in a warm car.
- Avoid drinking liquids from Styrofoam cups.
- Use glass or ceramic to heat or store foods.
- Use laundry and dish detergents with fewer chemicals, such as natural or organic products.
- Use organic soap and toothpaste. (Avoid fluoride.)
- Take nutritional supplementation necessary to off-set the estrogen and the estrogen mimickers: magnesium, zinc, vitamin B complex, vitamin E, DIM, and Myomin.

PANCREAS

The pancreas secretes insulin. Insulin controls blood sugar and is considered a fat-storing hormone. It is impossible to live without insulin, but we could live a lot longer and have a better quality of life if we had less insulin flowing through our bodies.

When we eat high-glycemic sugary carbohydrates without proteins, fats, and fiber, the pancreas responds by secreting more insulin than the body needs for health, longevity, and fat loss. Many of us suffer by having an excessive amount of this hormone, which causes the free carbohydrates in the bloodstream to be converted into fat. This fat is distributed through-out the body, mainly around the hips, gluts, and abdominal area.

When the pancreas is constantly assaulted by high-glycemic, sugary carbohydrates, it releases large amounts of insulin. The body eventually becomes insulin resistant or desensitized to the insulin. This condition is called type II diabetes. If you are suffering from massive releases of insulin, you will be happy to know there is a scientific way to eat more calories and decrease insulin secretion, along with decreasing body fat.

The Faith & Fat Loss eating plan allows you to eat more calories while decreasing body fat. It also enables you to stabilize blood-sugar levels by eating proper combinations, and eating 5-6 small meals per day. A rule of thumb in stabilizing blood sugar, lowering insulin secretion, and decreasing body fat is to **never eat a carbohydrate alone.**

Chromium is a mineral that helps decrease the amount of insulin necessary to stabilize the blood sugar. The reduced secretion of insulin, because of the presence of chromium, also reduces the conversion of triglycerides to be stored as body fat.

Adrenal Glands

The adrenals are two pyramid-shaped glands at the top of the kidneys. These glands secrete the necessary hormones of adrenaline and cortisol. The primary function of these hormones is survival. In extreme circumstances, and under stress, these hormones cause a fight-or-flight response, producing a tremendous amount of aggressive energy to attack or escape from a situation. Most people today have more mental and emotional stress compared to physical activity, so high levels of cortisol and adrenaline are not necessary to perform daily tasks.

Cortisol in today's society has been proven to be one of the hidden culprits of increased body fat; in other words, excessive amounts of cortisol will make you fat. Cortisol has many functions, but is often referred to as a fat-storing, muscle-wasting, stress hormone. When this hormone is released on a constant basis, it can decrease muscle size while increasing body fat.

When cortisol is released into the bloodstream, it converts glycogen (sugar stored in the muscle), fats, and proteins into energy. This conversion process causes a breakdown of the muscle tissue, thus decreasing muscle size and weakening the joints. If this extra energy is not used, the converted glycogen, fats, and proteins will not be replenished in the muscle and joints; instead, it will be converted into fat and stored in the fat cells, mainly around the belly and midsection.

Cortisol is released in times of stress. Ongoing stress, when not properly dealt with, causes a decrease of muscle and an increase of body fat. Underlying low levels of stress cause cortisol to slowly but consistently seep into the system, which makes fat loss harder to achieve. These stresses can be as simple as lack of organization, not completing projects, and procrastination, or as complicated as a deep-seated spiritual issue (discussed in the next chapter, "Soul Wounds"). Our objective, through a comprehensive plan, is to manage the spiritual, emotional, mental, and physical stress in our complicated lives in order to decrease the release of this muscle-wasting, fat-storing hormone.

Adrenal fatigue or burnout also contributes to the problem of excess body fat. A high percentage of Americans suffer with adrenal fatigue because of high levels of emotional and mental stress, lack of adequate sleep, and lack of endorphin-stimulating physical activity. Certain foods (refined sugars, alcohol, and other toxins) create additional stress. The body is resilient and capable of recovering from and adapting to stressful situations. But without proper nutrition, supplementation, and rest, the bombardment of long-term stress eventually breaks down the body's defenses and begins to burn out the adrenal glands. Once this takes place, the body produces additional estrogen, which causes an increase in body fat. Adrenal fatigue also causes a drop in blood-sugar levels, causing insatiable cravings for unhealthy and fattening foods.

Recovery from adrenal burnout is possible. Depending on how severe the burnout is, healing can take up to two years. The road to recovery requires a change in nutritional regimen, proper sleep, good supplementation, and detoxification. Most foods today lack the nutrients necessary for adrenal health, due to soil depletion. The following is a list of vitamins and nutrients necessary for adrenal health: B-complex vitamins; vitamins A, C, and E; manganese; zinc; chromium; magnesium; selenium; and Eleutherococcus Senticosus.

During this time of healing it is also necessary to nurture your emotional and spiritual health.

"ASK AND YOU SHALL RECEIVE"

You are probably surprised by the many different ways that an unhealthy over-stressed endocrine system can cause you to become overweight or obese. Our objective is to eliminate as many of these existing conditions as possible. We have discussed the role of stress and its ability to cause excess body fat. Some forms of stress are in our control; others are not.

As long as these stressful circumstances exist in our lives they will tax the endocrine system. God never intended for us to live in an obesigenic, highly stressful environment. But He has made provision for us even in this circumstance. Our greatest conciliation is that we can always go to our heavenly Father. He has the answer to every dilemma we may face. The Bible tells us to *"cast our cares on Him, because He cares for us {1 Peter 5:7}."* There is no problem God cannot solve through prayer. Allow Him to help you overcome the stresses in every area of your life and to direct you through complete recovery of the damage prior stress has caused your endocrine system.

God's Word says, *"You have not, because you ask not {James 4:2}."* Your responsibility is to ask earnestly, with a desire for God to fulfill what you are asking Him for. It is evident, if you are reading this book, that there is sincerity in your heart to achieve permanent fat loss. Let's take a moment and ask:

Dear God, Your Word says where there are two or more gathered in Your name, You will be in their midst. You also said that if we would touch and agree on anything, You would give it to us. God, we are in agreement for permanent fat loss. We ask You for Your divine intervention. Our struggles, hindrances, and obstacles are not easy to overcome. But according to Your Word, with man it is impossible; but with God all things are possible.

Your Word also proclaims us to be over-comers. We receive the overcoming power of God in our lives by opening our hearts and allowing You to work through us. We thank and praise You. We receive the victory now, in Jesus' name. Amen.

Chapter 6

Soul Wounds

"Unto thee, O LORD, do I lift up my soul." —Psalm 25:1
"He restoreth my soul." —Psalm 23:3

Hindrances are mainly produced by natural circumstances we can overcome with accurate knowledge, God's help, and putting forth some effort. Soul wounds, on the other hand, emotionally cripple and disable their victims. They penetrate deep, affecting us mentally, emotionally, and spiritually. If you are overweight or obese, your struggle with excess body fat may be one that is rooted in the soul.

Soul wounds are caused by spiritual arrows directed at the heart of its victim. This damage causes a continual stumbling block that distorts the view of those who have been hurt, and makes them see themselves as a fraction of who they really are. These arrows come in various shapes and forms through relationships, experiences, and circumstances. Any hurtful experience can scar the soul and if not dealt with properly it will cast a dark shadow over the rest of your life.

Soul wounds are personal and deeply painful, which makes it difficult for some people to share them even with those closest to them. They are rooted in the innermost part of our being and some of us have been in this state for so long we have learned to accept our condition and live with a wounded soul. But these wounds will prevent you from becoming all that God intended. You don't have to live with the pain or the excess body fat that your soul wounds have caused. If this is your condition, I urge you to allow God to transform your life.

It is important for you to understand that the spiritual arrows that cause soul wounds have been engraved with an assignment – to convince you that you are less, and to make you think you can't when God says you can. If you are overweight and have a soul wound, ask yourself, "Could I overcome my weight problem on my own in six months?" Your answer without thought might be "yes," but if you are obese why haven't you taken the time to conquer obesity? Now ask yourself, "Could the Lord overcome my weight problem in six months?" The answer is, of course, a resounding "yes." The Word of God encourages you that you can do all things because Christ's power accomplishes the work through you. It also says that whatever you think of yourself is who you are {Proverbs 23:7}. If you think good of yourself, you are. If you think you can move mountains, you can. If you think you can overcome soul wounds and obesity, you will.

It has often been said that victory goes to the strong, but this does not mean human strength or willpower when it comes to fighting soul wounds and obesity. If you have been unsuccessfully fighting this battle alone, with your own knowledge and strength, you'll be relieved to know that victory comes through God's Word and His strength.

The first step in healing is to acknowledge the soul wounds you are suffering with. The next step is to realize that you cannot win this battle alone, especially in a broken and wounded condition.

A soldier going into battle needs to be properly trained and encouraged before he can conquer. He needs to be in a mental state of victory. To further his confidence, he must be healthy and vibrant. Sending a soldier into battle discouraged, unhealthy, and wounded would seal his defeat. If you're battling against excess body fat and carrying a soul wound, you have entered the battle discouraged, unhealthy, and wounded. The scenario of the wounded soldier is a parallel to what you are facing. God would not send you into battle in this condition. In order to be victorious over the excess body fat, you must be encouraged, confident, and healed from the soul wounds that keep you from being who God says you are. The Bible says in Romans 8:37, "*In all these things we are more than conquerors through Him that loved us.*" The key to making this Scripture effective is that last phrase. The victory comes "*through Him that loved us.*"

SPIRIT, BODY, AND SOUL

David says in Psalm 139:14, *"I will praise thee; for I am fearfully and wonderfully made."* When God made you, He put you together with care and precision. Do you realize how awesome you are? God says you are something to be marveled at.

Let's look at how God designed us. You can see in First Thessalonians 5:23 that we are comprised of three dimensions that work together in unison, *"I pray God your whole spirit and soul and body be preserved blameless."*

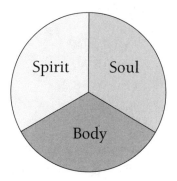

Man is a spirit who lives in a body and has a soul. Understanding this triune relationship of man will help us to better relate and deal with the soul wounds that find their way into our lives. Man as a triune being may be a truth that you have not explored. This truth is so important that there is a need to biblically detail what the Word of God has to say about this fact.

Genesis 1:27 states, *"God created man in His own image, in the image of God created He him; male and female created He them."* We are the only creation that God created like Himself.

God is a spirit {John 4:24}. God's image is found in the spirit of man, not in his physical body or physical appearance. If God's image was in man's physical body, we would have to ask ourselves what God looks like or better yet who He looks like. Is He five feet or six feet tall, black or white, male or female? My point is this, we can't all look like God physically, but we can carry His image spiritually.

Genesis 2:7 states, *"And the LORD God formed man of the dust of the ground, and breathed into his nostrils the breath of life; and man became a living soul."* In order to form something, you must first have material you can mold into the shape you desire. God created man in His image (a spirit), then He took the dust of the ground and formed man (a body), and then He breathed into his nostrils and man became a living being (a soul).

The Scriptures below further confirm that the three parts of man are individual, but at the same time they work together.

 Spirit   Body   Soul

Spirit	Body	Soul
Isaiah 26:9	Psalm 103:14	Psalm 19:7
Hebrews 4:12	Genesis 3:19	Proverbs 8:36
John 4:23-24	Genesis 18:27	Matthew 10:28
	Job 34:15	

There is a predetermined outcome for your body and your spirit. Your body returns to the dust from where it came and your spirit returns to God, but you determine what will happen to your soul. This is the reason the soul is the main target for the adversary. Pain and heartache are felt in the soul; decisions of commitment, loyalty, and integrity or lack thereof are made in the soul; and following your destiny is decided in the soul.

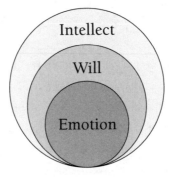

The soul is comprised of our intellect, will, and emotion which lives on eternally. When the soul has been hurt or damaged, we see life through our pain. This pain affects our direction and thought process. The negative thoughts that come from soul wounds generate negative feelings. Finally, these feelings manifest actions that prove the soul wounds exist. These soul wounds can only be healed by God's power.

CORTISOL

As mentioned in The Hormone Hindrance chapter, cortisol is a fat storing, muscle wasting, stress hormone. Cortisol is like a two-edged sword. It is necessary for proper functioning of the body, but it can be devastating if too much is released on a constant basis. Stressful circumstances, whether positive or negative, cause cortisol to be released into the bloodstream. Stress could stem from strenuous exercise, being caught in traffic jams, being overworked, or even lack of appropriate sleep.

Cortisol is released according to the amount and length of stress that is being experienced. It is naturally released at higher levels in the morning. When the body is under continuous stress, cortisol is released in high levels at inappropriate times. This causes the body to respond by converting muscle into energy, therefore creating high amounts of blood sugar that is converted into excess body fat and stored in the belly.

How does this fat-storing hormone affect you in everyday life? Below are two scenarios demonstrating the damaging effect of continual cortisol release:

Scenario #1

Mary had a six-month project that required a tremendous amount of time, mental effort, and physical work. She was not sure she could complete the task within the allotted time. Her sleep was disrupted throughout the night, and she consumed large amounts of sugary, caffeinated beverages to increase her energy levels.

In six months, Mary put on thirty pounds of body fat and her health had diminished. How did this happen? During the six months, the caffeinated beverages she consumed and her lack of sleep caused a release of cortisol. Her physically intensive labor and the mental stress of the task became more than she could handle, both of these stresses increased the release of cortisol in her system. And the pressure of the demanding time line caused more stress, which resulted in even higher levels of cortisol in her body. With an already slow metabolism and the excessive amount of cortisol – no wonder she put on thirty pounds of body fat.

Mary realized that she had gained weight because of stress, and she knew where the stress was coming from. She reasoned with herself that when this project was over, she would be relieved from the massive amounts of stress that had caused the release of the fat-storing, muscle-wasting stress hormone called cortisol.

The stress in this scenario would be considered a hindrance. The stress in the next scenario is a soul wound.

Prior to explaining the second scenario it is imperative to understand the role of the conscious and subconscious mind. The subconscious mind occupies 88 percent of the brain's capacity, while the conscious mind occupies only 12 percent. The subconscious remembers every event and conversation; it also registers every feeling and emotion. The subconscious plays a huge role in sustaining soul wounds.

The healing process of a soul wound is determined by how traumatic and deep it is, and how long it has been in existence. If a soul wound is acquired at a young age, the recording of this soul wound plays over and over in the depths of your subconscious mind. The effects range from minor to extremely severe.

Soul wounds often create feelings of stress that are irrational. You may have no recollection of why or how these feeling came about. You might not even realize that the past hurt is contributing to the suffering you are experiencing today. A wound of this kind will affect the rest of your life unless it is properly dealt with by God.

Keep in mind, stress triggers a release of excess cortisol into your system, regardless if the stress is derived from the conscious mind or the subconscious. Stress from festering soul wounds cause a constant dripping of cortisol for years and years, as long as the wound goes unhealed. This continuous release of extra cortisol causes the body to persistently add excess body fat, primarily stored in the belly.

This second scenario will shine light on how soul wounds remembered in the subconscious mind, along with a constant cortisol release derived from stress, will cause excess body fat.

Scenario #2

Julie's parents often let her uncle babysit her. From the time Julie was six until the age of twelve; her uncle violated and raped her. He threatened that if she told anyone he would hurt her family. Shame, embarrassment, and fear kept her silent. The violation committed against her caused her to fear and distrust all men.

Since her parents put her in this situation repetitively, Julie blamed them for not protecting her. This caused anger, distrust, hurt, and an enormous amount of insecurity. It also created a distance in her relationship with the two people she loved and trusted the most.

As she grew older, she became fearful of the dark and felt insecure in situations where she didn't have complete control. She became overly critical of herself and others, and extremely uncomfortable around men.

Julie trusted no one. Instead of talking to her parents or someone who she could trust in times of stress, she found comfort in being alone and eating what she considered to be "happy foods." These foods released endorphins and consisted mainly of fattening carbohydrates.

Julie became obese before the age of twenty-five. The soul wounds she encountered, beginning at the age of six, continued to affect her life because the soul wounds were not dealt with. Her early life started her on a path of a downward spiral. This one forced event changed the direction of Julie's entire life. The cortisol release caused by the mental and emotional stress in the conscious and subconscious mind turned what would be a completely fit, healthy, vibrant young woman into an unhealthy, sickly, obese woman. This whole subconscious process of releasing excess cortisol started with an early childhood rape. Julie had several other stress related factors stemming from the rape, which caused additional cortisol release. She blamed her parents for leaving her in this vulnerable situation and for not protecting her. This type of stress was not intended by God for this young child to suffer, so the body responded by releasing more cortisol.

Julie tried to replace the emptiness and loneliness she felt by developing a relationship with food that, at least, she could control…or so she thought. This addiction increased body fat two ways: one through the release of additional cortisol and the other through the fattening foods she ate.

As she got older, Julie became concerned about her excess body fat and started the cycle of fad dieting. This destroyed her metabolism, causing her to put on even more body fat. Through repeated bouts of depression and loneliness, she put on more weight, becoming hopeless and discouraged.

Julie's situation could not be solved by a diet or a fat-loss pill. Self-help solutions would never work for her. The core of Julie's problem was that she had stored within her subconscious mind a devastating, painful soul wound that could only be healed by God.

We can see from the two scenarios above that excess cortisol has an overwhelming impact on the lives of those who are plagued by a constant release into their bloodstream. This hormone alone can radically affect your whole life and it can create a battle against excess body fat that can't be won. To overcome obesity derived from excess cortisol caused by a soul wound, a true transformation is required. True transformation heals the spirit, body, and soul.

THE SOUL WOUNDS

A soul wound can come from hundreds of sources and be inflicted at any point in an individual's life. These wounds reduce the individual and leave them incapable of fulfilling their capacity. After a soul wound has been in existence for a long period of time, it becomes a part of our everyday life. For the most part, we consciously forget it until a trigger sets it off. But subconsciously it never leaves and the effects are constant.

When this type of wound is inflicted, it creates an emptiness in our soul so we never feel completely satisfied. We yearn for something more. We try to fill our yearnings with things like drugs, alcohol, sex, and comfort foods, which at best make us feel temporarily satisfied. When this euphoric feeling passes, we are left with a void that sends us on our next quest to fill the emptiness. These painful wounds may cause the development of unhealthy relationships with things or people, such as promiscuity, self-seclusion, or making compulsive purchases.

A common trait between a physical wound to the body and a soul wound is they naturally both desire to be healed. When you have a physical wound, given the right natural environment over a period of time, it will eventually heal. A soul wound, given a supernatural environment, will also heal. This environment is created in the presence of God. **God's desire for us is not only to face our soul wounds, but to allow Him to bring healing and comfort to our souls.**

Most people have one or more soul wounds, but few of us are courageous enough to face them. If your desire is to be whole and complete, take the advice of the apostle Paul and examine your soul.

If you examine your life and find traits that are unbalanced, you might be able to trace them back to a soul wound. If you know you have a soul wound in your past, you will probably notice the adverse effects of its existence in your life. It is not shameful to have a soul wound. The important thing is to address it and not allow its debilitating consequences to continue. Every soul wound has a different effect depending on our personalities, our level of tenderness, and the environments we grew up in. We may fail to realize soul wounds not only affect us, but they affect everyone close to us, including our children.

In order to more easily explain the nature of a soul wound I needed to find something they were comparable to. The best comparison I could come up with is that a soul wound is similar to a parasite. A parasite's nature is to survive. It camouflages itself so it can't be recognized, while slowly depleting life from its host. The same way a parasite deprives the body; a soul wound also deprives the soul. As long as the soul wound exists, life to the fullest cannot be accomplished.

Soul wounds can go undetected simply because some have been there so long that we have learned to live with them and they have become part of who we are. This makes it easy to deny we have a soul wound, but there are a number of things that can help us identify a soul wound in our lives. These negative characteristics have often been accepted as natural personality traits but, in all actuality, many of them are developed behaviors that stem from wounds to the soul. Here is a list of some common ones:

Lack of Confidence	Low self-esteem
Fear	Pride
Trying to prove yourself	Lies
Repeated failure	Sabotage
Denial	Insecurity
Unmerited anger	Hatred
Uncommitted in relationships	Depression
Addictions	Compulsion
Obsession	Promiscuity
Unforgiveness	Rebellion
Mental torment	Brokenness
Lack of trust	Rejection
Perfectionism	Withdrawn
Ashamed	Jealousy
Hardened heart	Coldness toward others
Self-destructive	Lack of discipline
Being **overweight or obese**	

If you have any of these traits, they could be linked to a soul wound. Many people who have these traits say, "This is who I am," "I have always responded like this," or "This is the way God made me." These are verbal excuses spoken out of a wounded soul. In all actuality, many times we deal with situations and relationships out of our soul wound – – not the reality of what is.

If you are struggling with soul wounds, you are not alone. They have played a part in many lives throughout history. Even King David, one of the great biblical heroes, suffered from soul wounds. In Psalm 88:3 he said, *"My soul is full of troubles."* David's son died as a result of his adulterous relationship. His wife was taken from him and given to another. His best friend, who saved his life, was killed in battle. A house of priests was killed for protecting him. He was banished by his father-in-law, the king, and left to live in caves. If this wasn't enough, his own beloved son tried to take his life. As you can see, David was well acquainted with troubles and wounds of the soul.

We are going to identify and explain just a few of the many soul wounds that commonly affect us today:

- Negative Words (Verbal abuse)
- Neglect
- Sexual molestation and Rape
- Childhood Abuse

NEGATIVE WORDS (VERBAL ABUSE)

Proverbs 18:21 says, "*Death and life are in the power of the tongue.*" Words are powerful.

In the beginning, when God created man, He created us in His image and in His likeness; in other words, He gave us some of His attributes. One of those attributes is the creative ability of words.

God spoke and said, "*Let there be light.*" Notice there was no light until words were spoken. Thought alone did not create light; it was only when the words were spoken that light came into existence. God gave us this same ability to create with our words. We can speak words of encouragement and watch a smile form on a loved one's face – that's power. Or we can say words that cause tears of sorrow that penetrate the heart and become a lasting soul wound.

James 3:1-11 tells us that even though the tongue is a small member of the body, it is very powerful and can be dangerous and detrimental if not controlled. What you say has the ability to inflict life changing soul wounds.

Humans learn by hearing something repetitively. In order to hear, words must first be spoken. In our formative years, negative words have the ability to wound and develop negative thoughts of who we are.

Throughout Scripture it was understood that an individual's name would be spoken to them more than any other word, so their name represented who they were and what they would become. In the Hebrew tradition, parents prayed prior to naming their children and God gave them names that suited the children's character. King David's name meant "beloved of God." One of his brothers was named Shammah, which meant "God is with us." Caleb's parents received his name from God, and it meant "one who is bold." Those who knew him referred to him as bold whenever they called him Caleb. The positive words we speak to our children form a thought process about who they are and who they will become.

Negative words can create deep emotional wounds that affect a person throughout his or her entire life. Normally, the people closest to you—your parents, spouse, friends, teachers, role models, and peers—are responsible for causing the deepest soul wounds because you respect them and take their words to heart. If you are told as a child that you are dumb, and you hear it often enough, it is possible you will become what was spoken to you. Few have the ability to rise above this; they are the exceptions.

If the words of others have convinced you that you will always be poor and never amount to anything, this can be a tremendous hurdle to overcome. Jeremiah was convinced by the negative words he heard repetitively that he could not speak on God's behalf. He felt fearful, insecure, and doubtful of his gifts and abilities. The only way the damaging environment that afflicted his soul could be reversed was through a positive thought process developed through positive words anointed by the Spirit of God {Jeremiah 1:4–6}.

Negative words not only affect us emotionally and mentally, but they have the ability to affect even our physical bodies. Suppose a mother talks constantly about her weight and how important it is for her to be skinny. Her daughter, who loves and respects her mother, wants to be just like her, so she begins to store these words in her subconscious. They begin to affect the way she eats and the way she views her own body. They have the ability to cause an eating disorder and a warped self-image. She could develop an anorexic or bulimic mentality, but within a few years she could easily become overweight or obese. This could be the result of decreasing calories, which leads to a slowed metabolism and abnormal metabolic functions. Due to the high levels of emotional and physical stress and her poor diet, she will experience an over-production of cortisol and insulin. The mother's words were not intended for her daughter, but for herself. However, when she spoke the words, her daughter heard them and embraced those same expectations for her own life causing a devastating soul wound. As you can see "*Death and Life*" was in the power of her mother's tongue.

A few years ago I met a young boy who carried thirty to forty pounds of excess body fat, a large amount of which was in his chest and stomach. He felt so insecure about his body image; he refused to change into gym clothes at school because he was afraid someone would see his flabby chest. One day he was standing with three friends when one of the girls said with the intention of making a joke, "You need a training bra." Those words destroyed him, and became a soul wound that continued to plague his life. The words of his friend were words of "*death.*" Even if he decreases the excess body fat, he will still have a problem with his body image because of the soul wound that was inflicted through the words that were spoken.

The words that have been spoken into your life, both positive and negative, have helped form who you are today. Negative words can cause emotional, mental, and physical stumbling blocks that can develop into life altering soul wounds.

NEGLECT

It has been said that actions speak louder than words. Negative words repeated time and time again can wound to the depths of the soul, but a single action can get the same job done instantly. On many occasions a word has to be repeated; whereas, an action paints a vivid picture that is understood immediately.

The definition of *neglect* is "to not give proper attention to, or a failure to care for appropriately, through carelessness." It can either be a single instance or a habitual lack of care. Neglect is more clearly seen when the attention or care is placed elsewhere; for example, a parent who gives more attention to one child and not enough to the other.

Most of us have felt neglected in some way at one point in our lives. Perhaps your father didn't attend a special function or event, such as a basketball game or dance recital. You could say this is neglect, since the attention that was desired was not given. But this is not the kind of neglect that causes lasting soul wounds; such as, a child being left for days without food and water. The parent not attending the child's function, compared to the child being left for days, is on opposite ends of the spectrum. One may leave a memory, but the other will leave a painful soul wound. The neglect that causes a soul wound has a damaging affect for years to come.

How deeply neglect affects an individual is determined by its frequency, duration, and severity. Neglect can affect our emotional and behavioral patterns as well as our spiritual, physical, and mental health.

In order to understand whether neglect has affected you, examine your past. The following are scenarios that show different types of neglect which leave scars. Although, we may not specifically cover the type of neglect you have experienced; this does not negate the pain, sorrow, or deep soul wounds derived from your experience. The pain of neglect shows no favoritism to its victim. Keep in mind; it is not limited to the examples below.

Sibling Favoritism

In the book of Genesis we read about twin boys, Esau and Jacob, who unfortunately lived in a dysfunctional home. It was well known that Esau was favored and loved over Jacob by Isaac, their father. Jacob knew that his brother had his father's heart. His father's neglect caused feelings of jealousy, rivalry, vindictiveness, inferiority, and insecurities that affected many areas of his life. The pain and damage Jacob experienced was irreparable until he allowed God to heal the soul wounds that resulted from his father's favoritism.

The story of Esau and Jacob has repeated itself throughout history with different families and under different circumstances. The adversary uses this form of neglect on a broad scale to create lasting soul wounds. Those who believe they are the least favored among their siblings often think,

What's wrong with me that caused my parents to love me less or to show me less attention? They might believe they are not good enough, smart enough, pretty enough, or just not any fun to be around. They may have negative thoughts toward their siblings, such as jealousy, rivalry, a desire to see them fail, or even, in extreme cases, to see them hurt or dead. And yet, deep down, they still love them. Many people end up hiding their pain because they are embarrassed. They can't express the negative feelings they have toward their siblings or their parents. Harboring the pain becomes the glue that keeps the soul wound intact, ensuring that it will continue to affect them into adulthood.

If you have a soul wound caused by this form of parental neglect, the effects will create a pattern that will transfer from your sibling to every relationship in your life, unless God intervenes. If you were neglected by your parents and didn't feel you were good enough for them, you may not feel good enough for your spouse, which could cause words and actions of sabotage. If you felt you weren't smart enough for your parents, you may develop a defeated mentality and never overcome life's obstacles to become your best. The other extreme is to become obsessive in your desire to prove yourself to be good enough. Neither extreme is healthy or productive.

The personality traits that are developed out of a soul wound become part of who you are. This makes it difficult to identify the soul wound and to acknowledge that it has affected you. After all, living under the influence of a soul wound is all you have ever known.

Spousal Neglect

This second scenario is very prevalent in our society. I know a lady who was dealing with overcoming soul wounds caused by neglect from her ex-husband. I'll call her Rachel. Rachel's marriage cost her fourteen years of her life. She said her husband always wanted what he couldn't have. He had an innate desire to hunt, pursue, and conquer. When they were dating, he said and did all the right things to get her, but once they were married she was no longer a challenge. So he sought out other women who he was not supposed to have. Rachel saw his eyes constantly wandering; this left her wondering, *What's wrong with me?* During the marriage she suffered the pain of finding out, time and time again, about his extra marital affairs. This relationship caused Rachel severe soul wounds. The soul wounds were a result of the neglect caused by him not wanting to spend time with her. He didn't make her feel secure, loved, wanted, or beautiful. He had very little desire for an intimate relationship or meaningful communication with her. He looked at and gave inappropriate attention to other women, and she constantly feared the next affair. These forms of neglect deeply scarred her soul and caused her to have low self-esteem, and feelings of insecurity and fear. Her situation made her feel she was less-than and that this was all she deserved. Her confidence and trust in men dwindled, and her heartbreak was so unbearable it felt like it was more than she could stand. The last of Rachel's self-esteem was destroyed when her husband divorced her for another woman. The soul wounds developed from this relationship caused Rachel constant stress, which contributed to her being overweight with abnormal belly fat due to the enormous amount of cortisol release. Because of the nature of her relationship, there were many soul wounds developed from her spousal neglect that she must deal with in order to be whole.

The soul wounds you may have encountered from neglect are not your fault, but you are responsible to appropriately deal with them. Regardless of how painful or deep your soul wound might be, there is no wound too painful or depth too deep that God can't reach down and lift you out of.

SEXUAL MOLESTATION AND RAPE

In a fraction of time, a single act of sexual abuse can sentence its victim to a life of turmoil and suffering. When a person is sexually assaulted, the effects are devastating. This type of abuse causes a soul wound that can't be healed unless it is properly dealt with.

If you have encountered this type of soul wound, don't suppress it or allow others to make light of it. You were not designed to carry the stress and pain caused by sexual abuse. One of the blessings of having a relationship with God is knowing that you can trust Him and cast your cares on Him.

Sexual assault is one of the most painful, embarrassing, demoralizing, violating acts that could be committed against a person. Rape or sexual molestation should not be hidden, nor should you pretend it didn't happen. You may think it is hidden, but the effects are evident in your feelings and behavior. Your own body becomes an outward expression of your inward turmoil. This violation of your body, mind, and soul will continually affect you, perhaps more than you realize, until you deal with it.

Rape and sexual molestation cause a lack of trust in people, including spouses, parents, teachers, and even pastors and priests. It can even cause a lack of trust in God. The biggest problem with not trusting God is that He is the only one who can truly heal a soul wound derived from abuse. Without the Lord, you are left to seek other means of deliverance, such as trying to suppress the pain, self-help, positive thinking, and hypnosis. These are all feeble attempts to accomplish what only God can do. When your attempts fail, you are left discouraged, depressed, and perhaps even suicidal.

A biblical example of the effects of rape can be found in Second Samuel 13. Tamar was a beautiful young girl who was raped by her brother. She expressed to him how shameful it would be if he raped her, and begged for him not to force himself on her, seeing that he was stronger than she was.

In those days, young girls wore colorful garments representing their vibrancy and their virginity which was the most precious commodity they possessed. To lose her virginity through any means other than marriage was a tremendous desecration and, in her eyes, destroyed her value, her importance, her self-esteem, and her ability to give this one-time gift to the man she loved and intended to spend the rest of her life and eternity with.

After Tamar was raped, she hid herself and covered her face and became depressed, reclusive, and withdrawn. The Bible tells us about Tamar's emotional and mental condition after the rape. In this modern era we are not only struggling with the mental and emotional, but also the physical effects of sexual abuse. Statistically, studies show that people who have been raped or molested have a greater tendency to become overweight or obese, and they struggle with body image. These victims seem to develop unhealthy relationships with food. They develop addictions out of a need for comfort or control. They long to satisfy the void they feel in their soul. So they eat and eat, eventually becoming overweight and obese.

Many chemically altered foods available today dramatically affect the pleasure center in the brain. These foods release endorphins that are considered "happy hormones" because they make a person feel good. Depressed victims of molestation and rape desire these foods because they provide a sense of well-being. Although they only get a temporary high from eating these foods, they are left with a craving to experience this high again and again, so they repetitively eat foods that are fattening and addictive because they satisfy this desire.

The foods we choose to eat are within our control. We now understand that the foods we are craving give us a type of euphoria. We also understand that these same foods create excess body fat, but because they make us feel good we want to continue to eat them. This creates a dilemma – – we want to feel good, but we don't want to be fat.

For years after an experience of sexual molestation or rape, subconscious stress will continue causing cortisol to be released in your system. Due to excess cortisol released in the bloodstream, excess body fat is inevitable. Understand this, once you put on extra body fat and slow down your metabolism the problem becomes more intensified.

You need more than willpower and desire to overcome this kind of soul wound and get rid of your excess body fat. You need God's help. He alone has the cure.

CHILDHOOD ABUSE

Throughout life we have many experiences—some good, some bad.

If you encounter circumstances that create soul wounds and they are not dealt with they will leave lasting scars that will stunt your growth and keep you from reaching your complete development and full potential.

Soul wounds can be inflicted at any point in life, but the soul wounds encountered during childhood are the most damaging for the following reasons:

❖ **The most formative years of your life take place during childhood.** If you were assaulted as a child when your personality was being formed, it will be difficult for you to determine whether some of your personality traits came out of the soul wound or if they were God's original intention. Insecurities can develop out of a childhood soul wound. For example, you may have been born with a God-given gift to speak, but during your formative years you were verbally abused by being aggressively told repetitively that you were dumb and had nothing to say that was worth listening to. Out of this insecurity, you found comfort in keeping silent. As an adult, you will fight against the gift and give the excuse that I don't speak in front of people because "I'm just naturally shy," "I am conservative," or "That's not my gift." Unless the soul wound is healed, you will never develop and use this God-given gift.

❖ **Children are limited in their ability to clearly express feelings and emotions partially because they have not matured in their cognitive skills.** Children are not mentally or emotionally equipped to reason with circumstances they are exposed to. As adults, we can reason out situations and consciously place the hurt and blame where it belongs. But as a child the hurt is internalized, creating a soul wound. If not completely resolved, it will be hidden in the subconscious mind and continue to have a negative, painful, counterproductive impact throughout the individual's life.

❖ **Soul wounds inflicted on a child are more difficult to deal with because the roots are deeper and interwoven into who they are.** We read in Mark 9:21-23, *"How long has this been happening?' Jesus asked the boy's father. He replied, 'Since he was a little boy. The spirit often throws him into the fire or into water, trying to kill him. Have mercy on us and help us, if you can.' Jesus asked, 'What do you mean, If I can? Anything is possible if a person believes.'"* Jesus asked the boy's father how long he had been in this condition. He asked this question partly because He understood that dealing with a soul wound derived from childhood is more difficult. The only way this boy could be healed was the Lord Himself had to set him free.

Childhood soul wounds have lasting repercussions that are intertwined with our personalities. They can cause a person to have unwarranted fears, insecurities, a controlling personality, anger, aggressive behavior, promiscuity, shyness, lack of trust, low self-esteem, etc. These negative personality traits interfere with our relationships with others and how we feel about ourselves. They can manifest themselves in our physical appearance, such as posture, facial expressions, attire, and, last but not least, our weight.

There is a definite link between obesity and childhood soul wounds. The underlying stress created by a soul wound causes an increase of cortisol release, which results in an increase of body fat. Add to that decreased physical exercise and poor nutrition, and this person will become seriously overweight. In time, he or she will likely become obese, unhealthy, and die an untimely death.

If you are overweight or obese and have a soul wound, you have discovered that your struggle with excess body fat is actually a symptom of a much deeper problem that is rooted in the soul. Superficial solutions—such as self-help books or programs, positive-thinking seminars, motivational tactics, or so-called holistic gurus—will only lead to a dead end and leave your soul wanting. A soul wound cannot heal on its own. To effectively overcome a soul wound, you need God.

If you or a loved one are facing some of the painful circumstances discussed in this chapter, I hope your heart has been opened to allowing God to completely heal you. If so, I would like to share the following prayer with you.

Lord God,

I come before You on behalf of the person who is reading this book right now. I ask in the name of Jesus that You would begin the process of a deep healing in their soul by reversing the effects of neglect, negative words, childhood abuse, and, last but not least and the most painful, rape and sexual molestation. God, I pray that You would reach down right now and give them peace and encouragement to try one more time. Let them know they are not a bad person, they have simply experienced a bad situation. They have become a product of their environment. They have been exposed to events that were not in Your original plan for their lives. Teach them that all things work together for the good to those who love You and are called according to Your purpose and that somehow the neglect will work together for their good. The negative words spoken over them, will work together for their good and even the rape or sexual molestation, must somehow work together for their good. Lord, if it requires for You to give them a miracle – You are a God of Your Word. We thank You and trust in Your precious promises. In Jesus' name. Amen.

Chapter 7

SOUL SURVIVOR

"I am poor and needy, and my heart is wounded within me."
—Psalm 109:22

Being overweight or obese is not caused by a single factor. As you have learned in the previous chapters there are many causes of excess body fat, and that without discovering the root cause it is hard, to impossible, to lose the extra pounds for any length of time. If you have come to the realization that you have a soul wound, and you are overweight, you can guarantee your soul wound contributes tremendously to the extra pounds you are carrying. In order to effectively decrease body fat permanently you must face the soul wounds and overcome them by turning to God with the understanding that His desire is to heal your soul. I am living proof that the Lord will help you overcome these deep wounds that continually hurt you and hinder your life.

The soul wounds that hindered my life may be a little different from yours, but the process of overcoming is the same. So allow me to share with you how I became victorious over the life-altering events that were intended to destroy God's purpose and any real happiness for my life.

Through all the years that I suffered with soul wounds, I lived a life of merely existing. I may have appeared normal on the outside. But on the inside pain, insecurity, and bondage controlled who I was, the decisions I made, and how I viewed life. By allowing God to heal the soul wounds, I began to thrive rather than just exist. I finally started living God's purpose for my life. In going through the process of allowing God to heal the wounds I had encountered, I became what I call a Soul Survivor.

A Soul Survivor realizes that the strength and ability to overcome comes from God. A Soul Survivor knows that God is the only one who can heal wounds to the soul. A Soul Survivor thrives, not just exists. A Soul Survivor has suffered and conquered deep sorrow, fear, and pain. A Soul Survivor learns to trust, believe in, and love others. A Soul Survivor truly forgives. A Soul Survivor develops peace and joy that can only come from God. A Soul Survivor knows the difference between change and true transformation. A Soul Survivor has transformed. I AM A SOUL SURVIVOR.

Psalm 109:22 states, *"I am poor and needy, and my heart is wounded within me."* In this verse, King David put himself in a position to be a Soul Survivor. In all his wealth and self-sufficiency, he admitted that he was poor and needy. The first thing David did was humble himself by acknowledging and admitting he was in need. David also confessed that his heart was wounded. Then David went to the only one who could heal the pain. He had a profound understanding that God specialized in healing broken hearts and wounded souls.

If you are struggling with a soul wound, coupled with being overweight or obese, until you become a Soul Survivor you will always be plagued with the hurt, shame, and extra pounds associated with the soul wound.

THE POINT OF CHANGE IN MY LIFE

A soul wound is like a bully. Until you put it in its proper place, it will continue to dominate and control your life. I know what it is to have a bully, called a soul wound, which continuously causes frustration, fear, emotional pain, and torment – – doubting that the circumstances will ever change. Part of the reason I am sharing how I overcame is to encourage you that you are not alone. If your desire is to be free, remember that the Bible says God is no respecter of persons. What He has done for me, He will do for you.

I had a painful start in life. Maybe you did too. But the most important thing is not how you start, but how you finish.

You had no influence over the country you were born in, who your parents were, or who your siblings were. You had no control over the perpetrator who caused a wound to your soul that continues to haunt you.

No matter how painful your beginning, if you give your soul wounds to God, you will finish in victory.

The soul wounds that were developed in my childhood followed me into adulthood, causing me to only trust in myself, which limited me from reaching my full capacity. I was so broken that a subconscious survival mechanism kicked in as a protection. Because of this I developed many unspoken rules that protected me from further damage. One was that I absolutely had no need for anybody or anything. These protective mechanisms and the unspoken rules outlining who I had become were difficult to prevail over because they involved my will, my conscious and subconscious mind, and my emotions. I had no desire to rock the boat or change by letting, what I would call, an intruder into my protected world. It was difficult for me to put my life in someone else's hands because I had no trust, not even in God.

A huge obstacle I had to overcome was admitting and expressing I had needs that only God could satisfy. As I developed a relationship with Him, I began, for the first time, trusting in someone besides myself. This was uncomfortable for me because I had created parameters around my heart to protect it from intruders who could cause hurt or pain. The four walls that were built around my heart were pride, fear, unforgiveness, and distrust. These walls kept anyone or anything from getting in; including love, good relationships, and most of all, the healing God wanted to administer.

Even though the soul wounds caused pain, the parameters or walls kept me in a place where the pain was at least tolerable and predictable. As long as I had the walls, nothing could further hurt me. I felt if there was one more painful incident or let down it would simply be unbearable. I chose to stay in a place where I felt I was in control. Later, I realized by trusting God what I thought would be unbearable He completely healed.

As my relationship with God deepened, I still struggled with believing the concepts of the Bible. I had many questions, like how the Bible could truthfully say, *"All things work together for the good to those who love Him (God)"* {Romans 8:28}. How could rape or child molestation work for my good? How could abandonment and the feelings and emotions that are too painful to put into words work for my good? How could insecurity, fear, physical and verbal abuse be good for me? What good could come from the deaths of my closest loved ones? These are some of the painful soul wounds and circumstances that God set me free from. I want to reiterate from experience that soul wounds are painful and hard for us to deal with, but they are easy for God to heal!

BREAKING DOWN THE WALLS

In order to completely experience freedom from the soul wounds that hindered my life, the walls of protection and bondage surrounding my heart had to be dismantled. The first wall to be brought down was the wall of pride. After it was gone I was able to admit I was in need of help. This was the doorway that allowed God to enter my life. By embracing humility, I started on my journey of being freed from the soul wounds that held on to my life for decades. I learned that in order for the Lord to come in and right the wrongs and heal the hurts, I had to welcome His help and admit I needed Him.

Another wall that needed to be broken down was fear. The nature of fear is to paralyze its victim stopping any advancement of thought, emotion, or forward movement. In order for me to move forward, I had to hate the fear brought about by my condition more than I feared the unknown.

The walls that were constructed around my heart did not allow any room for compassion or forgiveness. If someone let me down or disappointed me in any way, I immediately cut them off. There was no forgiveness or retribution for that person. These people, in my world, were no longer worthy of thought or emotion. This made it nearly impossible to develop any type of meaningful relationship. The wall of forgiveness had to be disassembled one brick at a time. The truth that helped me through this process was understanding that forgiveness was not only for the perpetrator, it was mainly for me. There was pain associated with the unforgiveness and as long as the unforgiveness remained, so did the pain. I forgave as much as I knew how, but I still felt the pain associated with the negative experiences from my past. Even though I desired with my whole heart to forgive, it was still not enough – the pain never left. The pain I had experienced was bigger than I was.

The best way for me to get this point across is by painting a picture you can relate to. Let's say a neighbor kid shoots your child in the back of his leg with a pellet gun. You examine your son and determine that he merely has a small bruise on his calf. This is fairly easy to forgive. Now let's say your son is playing in the front yard and a stranger drives by and shoots him with a shotgun and kills him. This stranger would be much harder to forgive than the child's friend. The first incident is within your capacity to forgive, but the second can only be forgiven through God's forgiveness working in your life.

Without God's presence in my life, I didn't have the ability to forgive those who so deeply hurt me. So I asked for God's help, praying something like this:

Lord, I have forgiven as much as I know how – to no avail. So I'm asking You to give me Your forgiveness for those who have deeply hurt me. Some would say just let it go, I tried that but it didn't work – the unforgiveness, hurt, and pain remains. God, if You can forgive all that was wrongfully done against You and Your Son, surely if I had Your forgiveness I could forgive what was done against me. So I'm asking You to give me Your ability to forgive. In Jesus' name. Amen.

As a result of this sincere prayer, God gave me His forgiveness.

My struggles didn't immediately leave. I had to develop a new thought process by having my mind renewed through God's presence in my life and his Word. I exchanged the comfort of the four walls that had surrounded my heart for the comfort of the Holy Spirit.

As I continued to cast my cares on Him, He proved how much He cared by healing my soul wounds. This developed trust, which gradually destroyed the wall of distrust. The unknown was not as fearful when I became more acquainted with God's love. For some people, healing from past hurts comes instantly. For me, it came in layers. I believe God is very capable of healing all of our pain instantly but, as for me, it was a process of learning to trust and forgive.

The Effects of a Soul Wound

Prior to knowing God, sin was a way of life for me. In my ignorance, I didn't even know that some of the actions in my life were sins in the sight of God. The adversary knows God hates sin. He fell from heaven and away from God because of sin. The adversary's desire is to reproduce his life of sin in us, so that we will fall away from God as well. One of the ways he accomplishes this is by creating soul wounds that bring about secondary sins and effects. Many of us have prided ourselves in keeping the Ten Commandments, not realizing that anything that hurts us, those around us, or our relationship with God is a sin.

There are three types of sin that we will be referring to. It is important to understand the kind of sin you're dealing with, so you can overcome it and place responsibility where it belongs. The three categories of sin are:

Original Sin – Original sin was inherited through the fall of man. Scripture states that all have sinned through Adam. {See Romans 3:23; 5:12–21}

Primary Sin – When we refer to a primary sin, we are referring to the sinful act committed and inflicted on a person that creates a soul wound in the victim's life. (Such as, neglect, verbal abuse, abandonment, rape & sexual molestation, etc.)

Secondary Sin – When we refer to a secondary sin, we are referring to sinful actions, thoughts, and emotions that are developed and expressed as a result of the primary sin (or a soul wound). (Such as, lying, pride, manipulation, adultery, pornography, etc.)

Note: Along with the secondary sin, you may also have additional effects, not necessarily considered to be sin, caused by the soul wound that hinders your life. (Such as, obesity, denial, comfort eating, sadness, sabotage, etc.)

God looks at the big picture and He loves us so much He wants to protect us from the repercussions of sin in our lives. Isaiah 1:18 says, *"Come now, and let us reason together, saith the LORD: though your sins be as scarlet, they shall be as white as snow."* God is saying to you and me, He is not hung up on our sin. Our sin can't change His love for us or His desire to be close to us. He knows everything there is to know about us, including our sins. As big as God is, He is saying to each of us individually that He loves us and sees the pain sin causes. To prevent further damage from sin, He wants to reason with us and come into an agreement wherein we give Him our lives which are stained and filled with sin. Then He will transform our lives, making us as pure and white as snow. God wants to alleviate the sin, so we can live out His complete plan for our lives. Jeremiah 29:11 says, *"For I know the plans I have for you,"* says the LORD. *"They are plans for good and not for disaster, to give you a future and a hope."*

As I examined all the sinful acts that were part of my life, I gained an understanding of where they came from. A significant percentage of the sin I was guilty of came from the "original sin of Adam" and not having a relationship with God. The remainder were developed out of the soul wounds: what I mean by this is sin begets sin. The illustration demonstrates if a sin was committed against you called a soul wound (or a primary sin), it is normally the root of several secondary sins and additional effects.

We want to explain God's view of the primary sin and how it affects you. Job 24:12 says, *"The soul of the wounded cry out; yet God does not charge them with wrong."* If you have a soul wound, this means sin has been inflicted on you without your consent. God hates the sin and pain that was caused in your life. He doesn't fault you for what someone did against you. God's desire for you is to give Him the primary sin that created the wound to your soul and allow Him to completely heal the pain and the effects that are attached to that wound.

The soul wound (or the primary sin) is a deep hidden sin rarely seen by others. For example, if you were raped as a child, few if any of the people around you know about it. But they do see the outward effects of the rape, and the secondary sins. These could include promiscuity (sin), lying (sin), insecurity (effect), or being **overweight or obese** (effect).

You may want to get rid of the secondary sins and the effects, but they can't be wished away. No self-help seminar can enable you to positively think them away. You need to understand there is no secret solution. Regardless of how much you understand the negative effects in your life, until you appropriately deal directly with the soul wound, the secondary sins and the effects will continue on their destructive path.

Most of the time, we try to alleviate the problem by dealing with the secondary sin or the effect. But we end up discouraged or irritated when the problem or the sin continues to resurface. Just like the dandelion. If you cut the flower from the stem it appears you have alleviated the problem, but within a few days the problem will recur. To get rid of the flower you must destroy the root. The root represents the soul wound (or the primary sin) that was inflicted on your life. The flower represents the effects, or the secondary sins, which stem from the soul wound (or the primary sin).

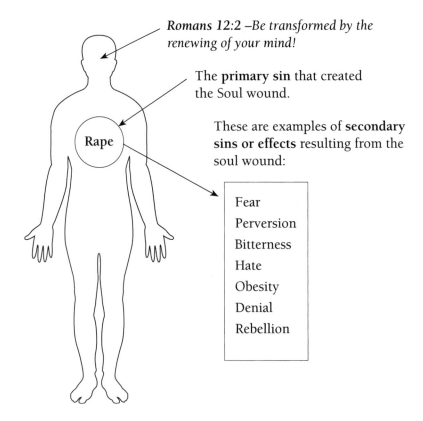

Romans 12:2 –Be transformed by the renewing of your mind!

The **primary sin** that created the Soul wound.

These are examples of **secondary sins or effects** resulting from the soul wound:

Rape

Fear

Perversion

Bitterness

Hate

Obesity

Denial

Rebellion

We have included an exercise for you to examine your life, so you can identify and acknowledge the soul wounds, the secondary sins, and the effects. This will help you complete the healing process. **The exercise can be found in the back of the book as Exhibit 2.**

A simple way to determine if you have a soul wound is to track the secondary sins or the effects in your life back to the source; it will lead you directly to the soul wound. Following is a short list of secondary sins and the effects caused by soul wounds:

SECONDARY SINS OR THE EFFECTS OF A SOUL WOUND

Distrust	Unforgiveness
Pride	Fear
Anger	Selfishness
Greed	Low Self-worth
Intolerance	Denial
Conniving	Feelings of inadequacy
Arrogance	Reclusive
Insecurity	Perfectionism
Low self-esteem	Sadness
Sense of betrayal	Depression
Procrastination	Self-pity
Bitterness	Jealousy
Rebellion	Inferiority complex
Doubt/unbelief	Excessive desire to please
Perversion	Stubbornness
Compulsive shopper	Anxiety
Lying	Manipulation
Compulsive hoarding (pack rat)	Judgmental
Guilt	Aggressive
Passive	Vengeful
Overly strict	Obsession
Loose	Compulsion
Immoral	Promiscuous

Brokenness	Impatience
Eating disorder	Comfort eater
Detachment disorder	Disfunctional relationships
Dissatisfaction	Discontentment
Drug abuse	Alcoholic
Self-destructive	Self-hatred
Overindulgence	Hopelessness
Controlling	Hate
Rivalry	Sexual addiction
Pedophilia	Loneliness
Pornography	Worrier
Grief	Adulterous
Violent	Vanity
Verbally abusive	Physically abusive
Emotionally abusive	Self-sabotage
Overweight	**Obese**

Soul wounds hinder our lives and remain deep within us for several reasons; including shame, fear, denial, and lack of knowledge. We can't take responsibility for the sin that was committed against us, but we are responsible for getting rid of the soul wounds that have come about as a result of those sins. Once we get rid of the soul wounds, we are well on our way to being a Soul Survivor.

I now realize that all the pain, torment, and suffering I went through growing up was necessary for the boy to become the man that I am today. God didn't cause the soul wounds or any of the hurtful events that took place in my life, but in His great love and power He made them all work out for my good. As Joseph said to his brothers, What you meant for evil, God turned it around for the good {Genesis 50:20}. Because of what God has done in my life, I have been truly transformed and I AM A SOUL SUR-VIVOR.

Soul Surviving Through the Five REs

I learned several things as I went through the process of becoming a Soul Survivor. I call these the Five REs of Soul Surviving ("Re" is the prefix which means to do over). The REs are the step-by-step process we are capable of doing that provide an atmosphere for God to do what we are incapable of doing, which is completing true transformation. The REs are the process you must go through to overcome soul wounds — while you are being healed physically, emotionally, and spiritually.

The following is a five-step spiritual exercise. Each step is important in achieving transformation and must be taken with your whole heart. Each step must be taken very seriously, with a knowing that when the process is complete, your life will be transformed.

Step 1 – Recognize

To *recognize* is to view and assess a situation accurately. Through self-examination, you acknowledge the soul wounds that continue to hinder your life. Sometimes it is hard to accurately examine and assess your own life, so we have included Exhibit 2 in the back of the book to help you through this process.

Step 2 – Renounce

Once you have *recognized* your soul wounds you must openly *renounce* them. This means to refuse or disown any association with the soul wound, proclaiming an outward rejection of its effects and influences on your life. For instance, if you were verbally abused, and this abuse caused you to harbor unforgiveness, hate, resentment, and pride, your outward declaration could be something like this:

*Lord God, I renounce the verbal abuse that I encountered. I reject all of its effects on my life, which includes hate, resentment, and pride. I choose by an act of **my will** to forgive the one who sinned against me. Thank You for Your love and faithfulness. In Jesus' name. Amen.*

The most important thing about the REs is that each step must be taken with your whole heart.

Step 3 – Repent

Now that you have renounced the soul wound (or the primary sin), which you had no jurisdiction over; you cannot excuse the secondary sin, which you are completely responsible for. You must *repent* and pray the prayer of *repentance*. True *repentance* means to turn away from doing wrong and start doing what is right in the sight of God. *Repentance* is not saying, "I'm sorry," with the intention of continuing on the same path.

The prefix *re* – means "to do over or go back." *Pent* means "the highest state." To *repent* means to go back to God's original intent for your life.

With this in mind, please pray this prayer with me:

Lord God, Thank You for healing my soul wounds. I also thank you for allowing me to repent for the sins I have committed against You and those around me. I believe that with this prayer, and Your help, my healing and forgiveness will be complete. Thank You, Lord. In Jesus' name. Amen.

Step 4 – Renew

Romans 12:2 says, *"Be not conformed to this world, but be ye transformed by the renewing of your mind."* It is important to realize your part in transformation is the *renewing* of your mind, which is the natural side of transformation. God's part is to change your nature and heal your soul, which is the spiritual part of transformation. When you do your part, you can expect God to do His. Your part is to put on the mind of Christ, abandoning the old thought processes. This is done by absorbing the Word of God in study and prayer, which cleanses your old thought process. In Ephesians 5:26 we find that God's Word is a cleansing agent for the mind.

It is a scientific fact – the only way you can change a thought is with another thought. As we learned above, God did not leave it up to you on what thought to put in place of your old counter-productive thought process. He provided the answer for you in Scripture.

Step 5 – Receive

The final and most important step is learning to *receive* from God. Picture yourself as an infant in desperate need of your parents' love and provision, realizing without them you absolutely cannot sustain yourself. You look to your parents and expect your needs to be met, without any doubt or inhibitions. In the same manner as an infant looks to her parents, we can look to God expecting to *receive* complete deliverance and true transformation.

EXPERIENCE TRANSFORMATION

The Lord gave us these loving words in the book of Hebrews and Revelation: *Harden not your heart, when I knock let Me in.* Today, through the words of this book, God is knocking. My advice to you is open the door of your heart and allow Him to do what you are unable to do, which is to heal your soul wounds and destroy the secondary sins and the effects, transforming your life causing you to be a Soul Survivor.

Here are some of the benefits you can look forward to experiencing:

- Truly living life and not just existing
- Fully loving God and receiving His love
- Experiencing God's intention for your life
- True joy and happiness
- Peace that surpasses all understanding
- True contentment
- Deeper meaningful relationships
- Giving and receiving unconditional love
- Permanently losing excess body fat

The first chapter of this book teaches us the difference between being changed and truly transformed. God's intention for each of us is to go through a true transformation. Physically and spiritually, we must lay aside every weight and sin that threatens to distract us from discovering who we are and fulfilling God's purpose for our lives.

As you go through the transformation process, the physical and spiritual weight will decrease simultaneously. The reduction of your physical weight will be evident to all who see you; and within yourself you will feel a sense of peace and rejuvenation.

The reality is God wants to transform you more than you want to be transformed, but before you can overcome the excess weight, you must first believe it is possible. As your thought processes change, you will clearly recognize that the secular way to fat loss, at best, leads to small reversible changes. You will also learn that God is the only source of irreversible change.

In the book of Genesis, we find the life of Jacob as he is transformed to Israel. The name Jacob means "supplanter, underfoot, conniving, and liar." From a child, Jacob possessed all of these ungodly traits. This name represented who the man was, not who God intended him to be. God allowed a series of events to take place in Jacob's life so he could see himself for who he was. At that point, Jacob was ready to give his soul wounds to God and repent for the secondary sins that had been caused by his soul wounds.

The root of Jacob's soul wounds came from the fact that his father loved his brother instead of him. This created soul wounds of neglect, abandonment, and verbal abuse. The secondary sins and the effects that stemmed from the soul wounds were inadequacy, hatred, vengeance, anger, rivalry, jealousy, lying, manipulation, etc. It was necessary for Jacob to be stripped of everything, including his pride. Being stripped of pride caused him to embrace the Five REs of Soul Surviving.

Jacob was born to be Israel. When God saw Jacob, He didn't just see a man, He saw a nation. Before this nation could be formed, Jacob had to be transformed to Israel.

When God sees you, just like with Jacob, He sees the big picture of your life. But before His purpose can be accomplished, you too have to be transformed. {References – Genesis 25:28; 32:24-32}

When you have completed the five powerful life-changing steps of Soul Surviving, you will be like a caterpillar as he enters the cocoon. You have done your part by creating the right atmosphere for God to complete the process of true transformation. After God does what only He is capable of

doing, you will become like the butterfly that takes wings and flies away –
never to be the same again.

We hope this Chapter has touched your life and convinced you that
soul wounds, secondary sins, and the effects only have as much power as
you allow them to have. God will complete what He has started in your
life. The Bible tells us in Matthew 5:6, *"If you hunger and thirst after righteousness: you shall be filled."*

If your hunger is to be a Soul Survivor and to complete true transformation, I would like to offer you this prayer of faith for your success:

*Lord God, I come to You on behalf of my readers who hunger for true trans-
formation and to be Soul Survivors. We are not asking for man's ability, but we
are seeking your ability. God, with man, what we are asking for is impossible. We
have seen man's attempts fail time and time again, but with You, Lord, nothing
is impossible. Whatever it takes to complete this work, we commit it into Your
hands. This means no more obesity, but health and fat loss. This means no more
depression, but the joy of the Lord.*

*Lord, I commit my readers into Your hands. I thank You for healing them
physically, mentally, emotionally, and spiritually. Thank You for healing those
with heart problems, high blood pressure, diabetes, hormonal imbalances, adrenal
gland malfunction, and every ailment, especially those associated with obesity.*

*God, I ask You to touch their minds and heal any mental disorders. Help
them to see what you see, show them the light at the end of the tunnel and give
them the strength, the desire, and the ability to reach into the unknown and acquire true transformation. In Jesus' name. Amen.*

SECTION III

Understanding and Defeating the Enemy

Chapter 8

EATING:

from Genesis to Revelation

"Why spend your money on food that does not give you strength? Why pay for food that does you no good?" —**Isaiah 55:2**

Isn't it strange God knew thousands of years ago that we would be spending billions of dollars on food that does not give us strength and paying for food that does us no good? These foods actually contribute to depression, malnourishment, sickness, disease, and obesity.

God created food to nourish and strengthen our bodies, and designed it to be one of our many enjoyments. But the very thing He created for our benefit the adversary is using to our detriment. The enemy would like to see us shovel ourselves into an early grave with our spoons.

The problem begins when our relationship with food becomes detrimental to a healthy, wholesome life. When God created food He said it was good {Genesis 1:11}, but too much of a good thing becomes bad. How did we get in this situation? There is no simple answer to this question, but the truth of the matter is that our first parents, Adam and Eve, were deceived about how and what they were to eat, and most of us have fallen into the same pattern.

In this chapter, we will take a step-by-step journey from Genesis to Revelation, revealing how food has affected us in the past, how it affects us today, and how it will continue affecting us for generations to come. You will see that science and history confirm the biblical accounts of the physical and spiritual repercussions of what we put in our mouths. We will begin by examining the first account of man straying from God's original intent for food.

ADAM AND EVE

Adam consciously ate the forbidden fruit, knowing it was detrimental to his health. How many times have you thought, *I want to decrease body fat and become healthier, so I shouldn't be drinking this soft drink or eating these potato chips?* After indulging, you are left with a feeling of disappointment and dissatisfaction, wishing you had never put that unhealthy, fattening stuff in your mouth. That's how Adam felt after he ate the forbidden fruit.

Eve's experience was a bit different. Satan convinced her to eat something she was directed by God, through Adam, not to partake of. She ate what was detrimental to her health because she was led to believe it would produce positive results. Many of us today embrace fad diets with the same thinking.

Eve's first mistake was failing to consult God concerning the nutrition that would be most beneficial to her. Most of us have overlooked the possibility that God has the answer to our nutritional and fat loss needs.

Eve's second mistake was listening to a voice that contradicted God's guidelines. How many of us have listened to such a voice, whether it came from a book, a friend, an infomercial, or some other form of media?

Adam knew that eating the forbidden fruit would produce negative results, but Eve was enticed, deceived, and misled. Genesis 3:4–6 tells us how it happened:

The serpent said unto the woman, ye shall not surely die: For God doth know that in the day ye eat thereof, then your eyes shall be opened, and ye shall be as gods, knowing good and evil. And when the woman saw that the tree was good for food, and that it was pleasant to the eyes, and a tree to be desired to make one wise, she took of the fruit thereof, and did eat, and also gave unto her husband with her; and he did eat.

God gave us five senses (hearing, seeing, touching, smelling, and tasting) for our safety and survival. When outside sources manipulate our senses, our safety is threatened and our survival becomes endangered.

Satan used these natural senses against Eve. Here is how the adversary enticed her:

Hearing - Satan first got Eve's attention through a luring conversation. He used her sense of hearing and convinced her that it would be to her benefit to eat what God had deemed to be harmful. How many times have you been deceived by an advertising scheme for some diet that sounded good, but did not produce results?

Seeing - Eve saw something that was pleasant to her eyes. Regardless of how good or bad a product is, if it looks appealing it has a better chance of being successful. This is accomplished by using pleasing colors, desirable settings, and tempting situations. We are enticed by how we feel when we see these advertisements. The intention is for us to see ourselves in these unrealistic situations; such as, becoming fit by taking a pill or decreasing body fat while sitting on the couch eating buttered popcorn, pizza, and ice cream. Eve experienced this because she pictured herself achieving something that was not attainable by eating what was advertised to her. Like Eve, after the convincing sales pitch, we experience a rude awakening.

Touching - In order for the forbidden fruit to get from the tree into Eve's possession, her touch was required. Once she touched the fruit there was a deeper attachment. This is a highly successful marketing technique. Once a product has been touched, the consumer experiences a sense of ownership. When you hold food in your hand that is unhealthy, yet enticing, what are the chances that you will decide not to eat it?

Smelling - As Eve held the forbidden fruit in her hand, she couldn't help but smell it. It must have smelled wonderful, possibly making her mouth water with anticipation. How often have you been tempted to eat something you knew was unhealthy simply by inhaling its pleasant aroma?

Tasting - Once we are emotionally attached through hearing, seeing, touching, and smelling our minds will be convinced to taste – just as Eve did.

This same technique is used today and we are equally affected by its progression. An example of this is when a car dealer first talks to you and gives you a great sales pitch (hearing). Then he shows you a car that is pleasing to the eyes (sight). The next step is to get you to sit in it, hold the steering wheel, take the keys in hand, and go for a test drive (touch). You take in that new-car scent (smell). You feel a sense of ownership. That moment is the greatest opportunity for a sale.

The five senses are the keys to emotional selling. It worked in Adam and Eve's day and it's clear that these same tactics are effective today. Not only does God teach us what we should and shouldn't eat, He also teaches us and warns us that the <u>adversary's tactics</u> are used in <u>advertising schemes</u> and deceptive marketing. Advertisement is not negative in itself; but when used to lure, entice, trick, and deceive you into a purchase which does not produce the benefits promised then it's connected with the word adversary. We must be able to discern the difference between a false advertisement that leads to our detriment, and a good one intended for our benefit.

If we continuously buy into the deceptive marketing tactics that do not produce the results promised we become desensitized and disheartened. When a good product comes along that meets our needs and desires, we are skeptical because of the disappointments of previous purchases. We have seen fat loss programs, diet supplements, and exercise equipment advertised using a very fit celebrity promising that within a short period of time you can have bulging biceps, ripped abdominals, and firm buttocks. After the purchase and within that short period of time promised you obtain no results; on the contrary, you are left with great discouragement.

Scripture makes it very clear; Adam and Eve each had a different thought process concerning eating the forbidden fruit. They set a pattern relating to eating, which has been consistent throughout history. Adam and Eve were instructed by God concerning what they should eat. They made an unhealthy decision to eat what God said not to eat, which led to their demise. We make the same decisions today by eating things that are unhealthy and dangerous to our well-being.

If Adam and Eve would have accepted the instruction that came from God, the results would have been different for all mankind. If we embrace God's instruction concerning what we put in our mouths, we will no longer suffer with being overweight or struggle with obesity-related problems.

ESAU AND JACOB

Esau worked in the field. When he came in from a day's work, he was hungry; it appeared he hadn't eaten all day. On his way home, he saw his brother Jacob making bread and soup and asked him to give him some. Apparently, he didn't have enough self-control or discipline to wait until he got home to eat. He felt it was necessary to eat immediately!

His brother made a bargain with him. Genesis 25:30–31 says, *"Esau said to Jacob, Feed me, I pray thee, with that same red pottage; for I am faint: ... And Jacob said, Sell me this day thy birthright."* Esau traded his birthright for a bowl of soup and a loaf of bread.

A birthright is any right or privilege to which a person is entitled by birth. Esau had a right to experience all the power, pleasure, and luxury his birthright allotted him. You and I have the same right to enjoy the fullness of our birthright, which includes a right to be healthy and fit. Esau forfeited his birthright by an unequal trade and many of us, by the same token, forfeit our birthright with an unequal trade. We find ourselves eating unhealthy foods, therefore creating an unhealthy body that leads to being overweight, obese, diseased, and having a shortened life expectancy. Esau understood the trade he was making, but he did not realize that his decision would have life-long repercussions. It is important to understand that the decisions we make either have long-term consequences or life-long benefits.

Can you imagine how Esau must have felt after he satisfied his hunger and realized he had forfeited his birthright for something so fleeting? He probably experienced depression, discouragement, even shame. These emotions are common in those who struggle with being overweight or obese because they feel they have no self-control or discipline. They are often ashamed of how others see them.

If you are experiencing these emotions and weaknesses, be encouraged. According to God's Word, you are in a good place. Once you acknowledge your weaknesses, God can come in and make a difference. In pride, we push God away. In humility, we draw Him near.

The apostle Paul became humble and allowed God to be his strength. This great man of God left these words for us in Philippians 4:13, *"I can do all things through Christ who strengthens me."* The strength Paul speaks of is available to you. You too can say, "I will overcome bad habits, food addictions, and being overweight or obese through Christ who gives me strength."

Enjoy your God-given birthright of being physically and spiritually whole, happy, and healthy.

THE CHILDREN OF ISRAEL

"We remember the fish, which we did eat in Egypt freely, the cucumbers, and the melons, and the leeks, and the onions and the garlic." (Numbers 11:5)

When the children of Israel went through the wilderness, they remembered what they'd eaten during their bondage in Egypt. They had been eating the same food for generations. Their taste buds had been trained to enjoy certain things, and they had no desire to change. Does this sound familiar?

Do you love the unhealthy foods you've been eating most of your life? Are you finding it difficult to change your daily menu? Do you enjoy the foods you're used to eating because your taste buds have become accustomed to them? If you have a desire to change, but can't get past the enjoyment of eating unhealthy, processed foods. You are in bondage.

God promised the children of Israel that He would deliver them from bondage. God has made that same promise to us.

The Lord also promised them a land they could dwell in that would become their own. In this land, He would erase the pain of their past and give them food that was delicious and nourishing. He desired to release them from any fond memories and attachments they had while in bondage.

Exodus 3:8 states, *"I am come down to deliver them out of the hand of the Egyptians, and to bring them up out of that land unto a good land and a large, unto a land flowing with milk and honey."* The Lord made a distinction between Egypt and the Promised Land. Egypt would be remembered as a land of bondage, fear, and suffering; this was associated with fish, leeks, and garlic. The land of Canaan was known for freedom and plenty; a land that flowed with milk and honey.

The children of Israel were in the wilderness because they had prayed for God to set them free. God answered their prayer by releasing them from the bondage of Egypt and bringing them into the wilderness. God's goal for His people was to escort them through that wilderness to a glorious land filled with blessings. But the children of Israel became disillusioned, discontented, and discouraged while in the wilderness because they failed to understand the meaning and importance of the journey, and they lacked trust in God to fulfill what He promised. They expected to go from point A (Egypt) and immediately arrive at point C (the Promised Land). But the journey enabled them to gain an understanding of the steps required to obtain their freedom. Without comprehending the principles of freedom, a return to bondage would be inevitable.

The bondage many of us face today is being trapped in unhealthy physical bodies. We want immediate freedom from this bondage. We want to jump instantly from being unhealthy and overweight to being fit and healthy. But we must go from point A, through point B, to achieve point C.

The time required to journey from point A to point C may take longer than you hoped. As you strive to achieve your fat-loss goals, you will experience many temptations to go back to your old way of eating. This is a period of discomfort, frustration, discouragement, and even doubting that your efforts will produce good results. But if you continue to seek the freedom God wants to give you, you will eventually arrive at the Promised Land, living in victory with an understanding of the process that was required, knowing that each step was necessary so that you never go back to where you were.

Once you have made up your mind to accept God's freedom and lose the excess body fat, you can enjoy the journey, being confident that God will help you every step of the way. Appreciate the small steps, knowing that each pound lost draws you closer to your goal. In this battle of the bulge, every pound you lose is a victory. If you continue to win the battles, ultimately you will win the war.

THE MAN OF GOD (ELI)

Eli was a priest, but he was undisciplined. His lack of discipline affected his eating habits and contributed to him being obese.

Eli's office required him to keep the light of the Lord lit continuously in the temple. First Samuel 3:3 says, *"Ere the lamp of God went out in the temple of the Lord."* This light represented God's shining on His people and His everlasting presence and protection. But Eli failed in his duties by allowing the light of the Lord to go out.

Eli had two sons who followed him in the priesthood. Because he failed to live according to the godly traditions that were passed down to him, his sons adopted his ungodly habits. The traits he passed down were lust, disobedience to God, lack of discipline, and overeating. The Lord became angry with Eli and reprimanded him for not having his house in order.

One way in which Eli dishonored God was by abusing the sacrificial offerings. Eli received the offerings from the people, then kept more than his share and ate it all himself. Eli clearly struggled with gluttony and became fat and unhealthy. First Samuel 3:2 states, *"It came to pass at that time, when Eli was laid down in his place, and his eyes began to wax dim, that he could not see."* Eli's eyes were dim; in other words, he was going blind. The Bible doesn't say Eli was diabetic, but diabetes is associated with being overweight and blindness.

Eli was a <u>heavy</u> man, and this was part of the reason he died. First Samuel 4:18 states, *"He fell from off his seat backward by the side of the gate, and his neck brake, and he died: for he was an old man, and <u>heavy</u>."* Eli fell over backward out of his chair and landed on his head, the pressure of his body weight coming down on his neck. His death was caused by a broken neck and his excess body fat cutting off his ability to breathe, thus suffocating him. His undisciplined lifestyle, including his overindulgence of food, affected him spiritually and physically, ultimately leading to his death.

We cannot take our health for granted just because we are not currently experiencing sickness or disease. Eli took his health for granted, not realizing that death would strike him suddenly. Early death is certain if we don't change our poor eating habits. Eli's bad habits cost him his life, and this lack of discipline also affected his children.

The Bible says, *"Train up a child in the way he should go."* {Proverbs 22:6} This is done by example. We need to lead our children in the right direction, not point them in the right direction. When it comes to healthy eating, our responsibility is to practice what we preach because our children will do as we do, not as we say.

More than 80 percent of overweight children come from families that have at least one overweight parent. Overweight children are at risk for serious health conditions like type 2 diabetes, high blood pressure, and high cholesterol, ailments that were once found only in adults. The emotional and mental effects of being an overweight child include depression and low self-esteem. These children are teased and picked-on by peers. They are usually the last to be chosen as teammates or playmates. Some of them end their pain by committing suicide.

If you want to prevent your child from becoming overweight or obese, ensure healthy practices that include proper nutrition, exercise, and healthy supplementation. Helping your children lead healthy lifestyles begins with you, the parent, leading by example.

SAMSON

Samson was noted as one of the strongest men in the Bible. But his character was a mixture of great strengths and great weaknesses. This combination is common in today's society.

We can examine Samson's strengths as well as the weaknesses that caused his downfall. By doing so, we can learn how to prevent the same misfortune in our own lives. In the desire to prevent our downfall, we must understand the nature of war and the devices of a true adversary. War can be described as a series of battles, strategically planned with the intention of conquering the enemy. An effective adversary analyzes his enemy; he looks at his strengths and weaknesses. An adversary's desire is to turn his enemy's strengths into weaknesses and to capitalize on his weaknesses with the plan of destroying him.

As the enemy analyzed Samson's life he could clearly see the following strengths:

> A godly upbringing
> Deep passion
> God's strength
> A strong will
> Leadership qualities
> Great faith in God
> God's favor

After the adversary examined Samson's strengths he then took note of his weaknesses:

> Disobedience
> Lack of self-control
> A strong sense of self-will
> Disrespect
> Lust for worldly pleasures, including food
> Dissatisfaction

Once the enemy compiled all of Samson's strengths and weaknesses, he used them to prepare a strategy to defeat him. The adversary has analyzed human behavior throughout history and learned that when the combination of lack of control, dissatisfaction, disobedience, and lust for worldly pleasures are present that this is the perfect environment to bring us into captivity. Food has been a perfect weapon for him to use against us and many times what we put in our mouth displays the negative characteristics listed above. We can see many of Samson's weaknesses by what he put in his mouth in Judges 14:8-9, *"...He turned aside to see the carcass of the lion. And behold, a swarm of bees and honey were in the carcass of the lion. He took some of it in his hands and went along, eating..."* As a Jewish Nazarite, Samson was commanded to keep strict vows. Some of the vows concerning food were that he was not to eat any unclean thing, nor touch or come near a dead carcass. Also, he was not to eat or drink from the vine. By eating from the carcass of the dead lion Samson showed his disobedience, dissatisfaction, worldly lust, and lack of self-control. By using these weaknesses the adversary was able to win a temporary victory over Samson's life.

In 2 Corinthians 13:5 Scripture says, *"Examine yourselves, whether ye be in the faith; prove your own selves..."* It is a godly thing to examine yourself to see if you are dissatisfied, disobedient, lacking in self-control, and lusting for worldly pleasures. If so, be assured the adversary has a plan for your demise. The adversary uses our strengths and our weaknesses against us to bring us into bondage. He has had victory in these battles long enough. It is time for us to take responsibility to win the war.

THE PARALLEL OF MASS DESTRUCTION AND FOOD

Mass destruction, in the Old Testament, represented the end for those who were involved. But before the kingdom of God is revealed mass destruction must have its place one last time. In Luke 17, as Jesus interacted with the Pharisees they asked a pressing question, *"When will the kingdom of God come?"* The Lord's response was that before His return there would be a final mass destruction. He let them know destruction comes when certain variables exist; which consists of sin, riotous living, and being out of control with food and drink. Whenever you see these variables, destruction is not far off. We are going to examine three major accounts of mass destruction and the involvement of food, as narrated by Jesus.

Luke 17:26-27,

(26)*As it was in the days of Noe, so shall it be also in the days of the Son of man.*

(27) *They did eat, they drank, they married wives, they were given in marriage, until the day that Noe entered into the ark, and the flood came, and destroyed them all.*

In the last days of Noah's generation overeating, drinking, and riotous living were vital signs of the end times. This demonstrated the people were out of control in many areas, including what they put in their mouths. Jesus said this is an indication of what will take place during the last days concerning us. The circumstances between the last days of Noah's generation and the last days prior to the return of Christ are identical concerning sin, riotous living, and being out of control with food and drink. The adversary has seen the struggle mankind has with food and uses it to our disadvantage, and capitalizes on it knowing that it was given to us from God for our pleasure. The issue we are dealing with today is excess body fat caused by having an unhealthy relationship with food. Ask yourself this question, "Am I out of control with my eating?" If the answer is "yes," God does not want you to be in bondage to food.

Let's look at the similarities between the days of Noah and the days of Lot. These two men were considered righteous because they were obedient to God. We notice they followed the instructions they were given. Noah was told to build an ark, and without hesitation he obeyed. Likewise, Lot was told to leave his home, all of his friends, and any worldly possessions he owned; and was instructed not to look back. He obeyed. What we see here are two men who were in tune with God and were willing to obey Him; while the rest had an unhealthy relationship with food and were consumed with riotous living, worldly pleasure, and disregard for the Word and the law of God. These are ungodly traits that the adversary is looking to capitalize on in every individual's life. We can see he is being very effective today.

Luke 17:28-30,

(28) Likewise also as it was in the days of Lot; they did eat, they drank, they bought, they sold, they planted, they builded;

(29) But the same day that Lot went out of Sodom it rained fire and brimstone from heaven, and destroyed them all.

(30) Even thus shall it be in the day when the Son of man is revealed.

Notice in the days of Noah and Lot, the adversary used what they put in their mouths to distract them. In Luke 21:33-36, Jesus prophesied that the food God intended to enhance health and longevity would be used against those in the last days who refuse to take heed to God's counsel. **The Lord gave us this warning which demands our attention, so we will not become a part of this ageless pattern and the statistic that is sure to come.**

Let's examine the words of Jesus in Luke 21:33-36,

(33) Heaven and earth shall pass away: but my words shall not pass away.

(34) And take <u>heed</u> to yourselves, lest at any time your <u>hearts</u> be <u>overcharged</u> with <u>surfeiting</u>, and <u>drunkenness</u>, and cares of this life, and so that day come upon you unawares.

(35) For as a snare shall it come on all them that dwell on the face of the whole earth.

(36) Watch ye therefore, and pray always, that ye may be accounted worthy to escape all these things that shall come to pass, and to stand before the Son of man.

In Verse 34, Jesus gives us a statement of warning. This verse is so significant that it deserves to be fully examined. Let's use the Greek translation to define several of the words in this passage, so we can fully understand what the Lord is revealing to us.

Heed (Greek *prosecho*): to pay attention to, to be cautious concerning, to apply oneself, to be aware of

Heart (Greek *kardia*): thoughts, feelings, and desires

Overcharged (Greek *baruno*): burdened, to be weighed down, heavy

Surfeit (Greek *kraipale*): to glut or to be gluttonous (overeating), debauch (to be drunk with food)

Drunkenness (Greek *methe*): intoxication

Now let's look at Luke 21:34 with the Greek definitions added:

Take heed (pay attention or be aware) to yourself lest at anytime your heart (your thoughts, feelings and desires) be overcharged (heavy burdened) with surfeiting (overeating and glutton; being out of control with food), and drunkenness (full of strong drink), and cares of this life and so that day (the coming of Christ) come upon you unawares.

Jesus explained to us three accounts of how food has been used against us in the past, how it is being used against us today, and how it will continue being used against us in the future. After our examination of the account in Luke 21, we can see the Lord is making an important declaration here concerning our relationship with food that we ought to pay attention to. The terrifying reality we are faced with is the fact that food has been used effectively, throughout the ages, against mankind. Jesus has brought it to the forefront, pleading with us to take heed. The fearful thing is that He spoke this, centuries ago, yet not many people have acknowledged the profound evidence, prophecy, and exhortation that has been given to us in Scripture. If this does not change, the statistics of being overweight and obese, along with sickness, disease, and death will continue to climb.

Two thousand years ago, Jesus said that in our day and age the majority of the population would be out of control with their eating. He revealed this to us as a friend. In John 15:15 Jesus states, *"I no longer call you slaves, because a master doesn't confide in his slaves. Now you are my friends, since I have told you everything the Father told me."* Let us take heed to what Jesus has revealed to us so we don't become part of man's massive downfall concerning food.

REVELATION

Genesis represents the beginning; Revelation represents the end. In Genesis, the adversary's plan was to destroy mankind by using food. His plan would have worked if God had not intervened, as He always does.

God intervened in the beginning with Adam and Eve and has continued doing so throughout history. But intervention after the fact is not God's best. His desire is for us to allow His Word to be the authority in our lives; then intervention won't be necessary.

The adversary's desire was to destroy Adam, which means mankind, he failed. Today he has developed another plan to destroy Adam, again Adam means mankind. In the beginning Adam represented two people; today Adam represents over six billion people.

In Luke 21:34, Jesus revealed the adversary's plan to use food against us. (Being overweight or obese has been doubling and tripling over the past three decades with no indication of slowing down and every indication of increasing.) For the adversary to be effective, he has to do with us what he did with Eve: cause us to doubt God's Word, to see it as irrelevant or unimportant, and to look to another resource to find the answers to our current situations; including, fat loss. In times past the people of God yielded to His intervention. Will you yield to the Lord's direction or to the adversary's plan to make you addicted to unhealthy, fattening, processed foods?

In the last book of the Bible, God has revealed to us what is to come. And in Philippians 3:19, the Apostle Paul said that many will allow their bellies to become their god. If you personally become Philippians 3:19, where your belly is your god, and then you collide with Revelation 13:16-18; let's view what this would look like:

Revelation 13:16-18,

(16) He causeth all, both small and great, rich and poor, free and bond, to receive a mark in their right hand, or in their foreheads:

(17) And that no man might buy or sell, save he that had the mark, or the name of the beast, or the number of his name.

(18) Here is wisdom. Let him that hath understanding count the number of the beast: for it is the number of a man; and his number is six hundred threescore and six.

In the last days, we will have no buying power without the mark of the beast. If your belly has become your god and you don't have the ability to buy, this means you won't be able to purchase food for yourselves or your loved ones. Up until this point, if God's Word has not been the governing authority in this area of your life, you will be forced to make a decision to please God. Your determination will become which one is your God — is it God Jehovah or god your belly?

Jesus, the Perfect Example

Jesus came to restore to us everything that was lost by the disobedience of our first parents, Adam. The first Adam {Genesis 5:2} failed because they were disobedient and doubted God's Word by eating the forbidden fruit. The second Adam, Jesus Christ {1 Corinthians 15:45}, overcame because He obeyed God by trusting in His Word, and refusing to eat and listen to the word's of doubt that came from the adversary.

Jesus understood the pleasure and pressure, as well as the positive and negative impact that food has had on the human race from the very beginning, and how it would continue to affect us throughout history. He knew His response to the adversary concerning food would be a lasting example of hope, so His followers could believe that it is possible to overcome the temptations that would be brought against us.

Luke 4:3-4 says, *"And the devil said unto Him, If thou be the Son of God, command this stone that it be made bread. And Jesus answered him, saying, It is written, that man shall not live by bread alone, but by every Word of God."* Jesus was tempted in an area that at least 70% of us have been affected by. He made a godly decision by looking to God's Word for the answer. If you are overweight or obese, this is your opportunity to identify with Christ and make a healthy decision by trusting God to give you the answer concerning food and fat loss.

Jesus is the perfect example for every area of life. We see Him exhibit the highest form of discipline by overcoming all worldly lusts.

He displayed complete self-control, even when He reached the place of absolute human weakness from fasting forty days (Luke 4:3–4). In spite of His need to eat in order to survive, He trusted in God's Word completely, even when those words were misrepresented to Him by Satan. Jesus responded to the adversary by quoting the word of God found in Deuteronomy 8:3.

Perhaps you think that because Jesus was the Christ, He wasn't tempted. But Hebrews 4:15 tells us, "*We have not a high priest which cannot be touched with the feeling of our infirmities; but was in all points <u>tempted like as we are</u>, yet without sin.*"

It is obvious that food has been an effective tool used against us by the adversary throughout history. Jesus proved, by His example, that we could overcome this attack by relying on God and trusting in His Word. The Lord gave us words of encouragement in John 16:33: "*These things I have spoken unto you, that in me ye might have peace. In the world ye shall have tribulation: but be of **good cheer**; I have overcome the world.*" Jesus is telling us, "I endured the same temptations you are dealing with. I know what it's like. But be of good cheer. I have overcome the world and I will help you do the same."

You may have struggled with food for so long it may seem impossible to overcome your impulses. But Jesus promised to help you so your struggle with food will not defeat you.

Chapter 9

FIGHTING AN ENEMY YOU LOVE

"Fight the good fight of faith." —*1 Timothy 6:12*

"And the Lord said unto him, surely I will be with thee."
—*Judges 6:16*

If you have been trying to decrease body fat, restore your health, and increase longevity, you are engaged in a fight. A fight to defend your God-given right to be healthy, fit, and lean. Even though you may not recognize the fight, the effects of this battle are evident. It can deplete your energy, increase your stress level, create a sense of failure, and make you feel overwhelmed.

The first step to winning the fight is acknowledging that there is a battle. But the thought of fighting an enemy isn't very appealing. Most of us have enough struggles. We deal with stressful situations every day, like balancing our careers, our families, and our personal obligations. On top of this, many struggle with food addictions, cravings, carrying excess body fat, being unhealthy, or feeling depressed. You may feel like your life is too busy to add something else, especially a fight.

To make matters worse, this fight appears to be against an enemy we love. This creates an inner conflict because we are pushing half the time and pulling half the time. This type of struggle ultimately ends in defeat because while half the time our efforts are focused on defeating the enemy, the rest of the time we are giving aid to the enemy. At the same time, the enemy focuses 100 percent of his efforts against us. His efforts added to our own, means that 150% is being used against us. In order to win the battle, we must decide that our opponent is indeed an enemy. This will end the inner conflict. Then we can give 100 percent of our efforts to being victorious.

An enemy is someone who engages in antagonistic activities against another. The desire of an enemy is to destroy and render his opponent helpless, without mercy. An enemy is to be respected, but also hated, feared, and kept at a distance.

When you love someone or something, your desire is to draw them close with a warm embrace and to watch over and protect them.

Fighting an enemy you love creates an internal struggle because your desire is to love and embrace, but at the same time to hate and push away. This dilemma makes it impossible to destroy the opposing force. Deep within we feel a tug-of-war, trying to fight an enemy we love.

DAVID'S BATTLE

King David could definitely relate to the concept of fighting an enemy he loved. David had a deep love for God and his family. He would have given anything for them, even his life. David's son Absalom was deeply loved by many citizens in the kingdom, but their love could not compare to the love his father, David, had for him. But as much as David loved his son, he hated his destructive behavior.

Absalom grew up to be disobedient, prideful, rebellious, and thought he should be king in David's place. Just as Lucifer had become disobedient, prideful, rebellious, and determined to take over God's throne. Absalom convinced many men to join him in his pursuit to dethrone the man who loved him most. During this conflict, Absalom even tried to kill his father.

This was a sad situation seeing that David loved his enemy. Joab, the captain of the army, stated to David with amazement in Second Samuel 19:6, "*Thou lovest thine enemies.*"

David sent out his army to defeat his son's army, but gave them strict orders not to touch the man Absalom. War was a way of life for David, and he was good at what he did. He knew how to fight and win. But this was a war David was not excited about fighting. Regardless of the outcome, he would be at a loss. A victory would mean the death of his son; a defeat would mean the loss of his own life and jeopardy to his kingdom. This was truly a lose-lose situation.

After the battle was fought and the war won, David had one question: *"What about the man Absalom?"* He asked this question several times, showing his deep concern for the enemy he loved. David finally heard the devastating news that almost sent him to his own death: Absalom, his son, was dead. David's devastation is shown vividly in Second Samuel 18:33:

> *The king was much moved, and went up to the chamber over the gate, and wept: and as he went, thus he said, O my son **Absalom**, my son, my son **Absalom**! would God I had died for thee, O **Absalom**, my son, my son!*

By David's example we can clearly see that it is nearly impossible to aggressively pursue, with the intention of destroying, an enemy we love.

REDEFINING THE ENEMY

Many people have a love-hate relationship with food that is similar to the relationship David had with his son. You love the pleasure and taste of food, but hate the excess body fat caused by overindulgence or having an inappropriate relationship with food. The problem is not your love for food because God created food for our enjoyment and for our nourishment.

Even in the ministry of Jesus, we notice that when the people were hungry He understood that it was important to sustain them by filling their stomachs before He was able to effectively fill their spirits. On many occasions Jesus sat down with his disciples and enjoyed the pleasures of food and fellowship.

Food has always been a part of social events. It is the centerpiece at most family and community gatherings, including church events, birthday parties, baby showers, holiday get-togethers, and casual fellowshipping with friends. God created us with an innate desire and love for food. Without this natural desire, eating would be a chore rather than a delight. Many of us might forget to eat, which would cause us to become malnourished and unhealthy, and quickly die. The fact is the desire for food is an innate part of who we are as human beings.

The problem is not our love for food, but our relationship with food and the difference between the foods we eat today versus the foods God created for us to eat. The Lord's original intention for food was to nourish and supply energy to sustain the body and give us long life. Today, much of what we consider to be food has very little nutrition, but high calories. Some foods are not only fattening, but highly toxic, even carcinogenic, decreasing our life expectancy. These so-called foods can also cause hormone imbalances that increase cravings and addictions.

This is where we seem to be conflicted, <u>we love food and we hate food at the same time</u>. We realize life is impossible without the consumption of food. We consider food to be both good and bad. Actually, the root cause of the problem goes much deeper.

PARALLEL BETWEEN ABSALOM AND FOOD

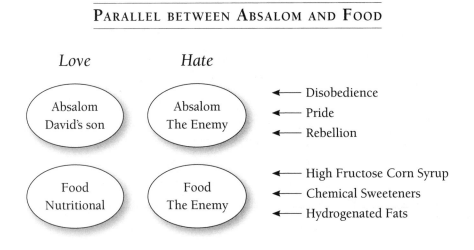

We can identify with the parallel between David's relationship with Absalom and our relationship with food when it comes to fighting an enemy we love. In the illustration above, we can see that God gave David a natural love for his son Absalom, just like God gave us a natural love for nourishing food. Like most parents, David saw the good in Absalom and knew his potential. But the negative course of events in Absalom's life caused him to change from being innocent to corrupt.

By the same token, when food was created, God Himself said it was good. When we eat nutritious foods, we have the potential of increasing our life span. But a large percentage of the food we consume has become unhealthy through a negative course of events throughout history. These changes are attributed to the food industry's manipulations under the subtle persuasion of the adversary.

Over time, Absalom developed the negative traits of disobedience, pride, and rebellion because of the adversary's influence in his life. Some of our foods, over the course of time, have become something that God never intended for them to be as well. Much of the foods today are contaminated, processed, and detrimental to our health. These foods have been changed by hydrogenation, the addition of high-fructose corn syrup, chemical sweeteners, etc.

Absalom and toxic foods, because of the influence of the adversary, are viewed as the enemy. David had an emotional bond with his son, and we emotionally bond with food. These deep bonds are developed early in life, making it nearly impossible for us to separate what we love from the enemy.

The True Enemy

The adversary wanted to destroy David and his kingdom, but to accomplish this he needed a door into David's life. Absalom became that door. The adversary also wants to destroy us. To do this he needs an open door. What better tool to use than food?

The enemy knows God made food pleasurable as well as necessary for our physical survival. Because most of us eat multiple times a day, the adversary has numerous opportunities daily to attack us using something we desire and love. As we learned in Eating from Genesis to Revelation, the adversary has effectively used food against us from the very beginning. There is a progression and an increase of intensity using food against us. This can be seen historically, biblically, scientifically, and also in the physical bodies of those around us.

Too often, we address what the eye can see instead of the root of the problem. But the root must be dealt with first in order to obtain lasting victory. We were created with a natural desire to ingest food. But the enemy, who is a spirit and can't be seen, has taken what God intended to be helpful and made it harmful.

What we have done is directed the battle at our food because we can see it, touch it, and taste it. But food itself is not the enemy.

THE DETERIORATION OF FOOD

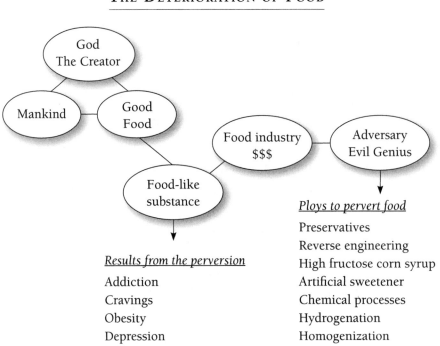

Results from the perversion

Addiction
Cravings
Obesity
Depression

Ploys to pervert food

Preservatives
Reverse engineering
High fructose corn syrup
Artificial sweetener
Chemical processes
Hydrogenation
Homogenization

The above illustration shows some of the steps used by the adversary to take food that was created to be good, healthy, and nutritious to a perverted state; which is unhealthy, filled with empty calories, and a cause of sickness and obesity.

God created food for the good of mankind. Man ate food and became healthy and energetic. But a lot of what we eat today is closer to a food-like substance, rather than food, because what we are eating does the exact opposite; it destroys our health and deprives us of energy. We have developed an affinity or love for these substances because they closely resemble the food that God originally created for us.

Some of the foods God created have deteriorated over time in such a way that it has been hard for us to see the change. For example, whole rolled oats are loaded with life-giving nutrition. But today's sweetened cereals are loaded with empty calories that contribute to obesity and associated ailments. These are both considered to be breakfast cereals and often times, with our busy schedules, it is easier to choose the sweetened cereal for its convenience not considering the long term implications of the choices we make.

At one time, consumers saw the process food went through firsthand, from the time it left the tree or the field until it was served at the dinner table. Today, we have very little knowledge of this process. It is amazing what has happened over the past thirty years. The food industry, which is a trillion-dollar industry controlled by money, has cut corners to make a higher profit. They cheapen and destroy good-quality foods to reduce the expense and increase shelf life, using toxic chemical processes, such as hormone and antibiotic injections, homogenization, hydrogenation, reverse engineering, artificial sweeteners, high-fructose corn syrup, MSG, and unhealthy preservatives, not to mention carcinogenic substances like pesticides, insecticides, and herbicides. Sixty five years ago we were not exposed to these life threatening chemicals and processes.

The adversary's plan is to negatively affect every human being on the planet with one sweep. How could he complete such a plan? What could he possibly use that is common to every human being in the world? Is there one thing that all of us need and have a natural love for? The answer to these questions is very simple – food. This is the tool that the adversary has used effectively and will continue to use.

Many of us have considered food to be our enemy using foolish means to fight this battle, including fad diets, only to find ourselves in worse shape. Others have pointed a finger at the food industry. But we cannot completely blame them for our condition. We must identify the true enemy; by doing so, this will allow us to completely embrace food and fight against the real enemy. The real culprit is the one who spoke to Eve in the garden and said, *"You shall not surely die."* The serpent has struck again. He is an evil genius who continues to influence what is happening to our food. By embracing the adversary's plan and purpose concerning food, we indirectly embrace him.

OUR BATTLE STRATEGY

The adversary has camouflaged himself well and is hidden behind the idea that food is the enemy. Now that we realize our love for food is God given, we should no longer feel guilty because we love food. Since our true enemy has been revealed, we can intelligently and aggressively fight him with the desire to be victorious. In order to be effective in this battle, we must understand our enemy and recognize his tactics. First Peter 5:8 says, *"Be sober, be vigilant; because your adversary the devil, as a roaring lion, walketh about, seeking whom he may devour."* And then we must know what it takes to defeat him. Second Corinthians 10:4 gives us insight on how to do this: *"For the weapons of our warfare are not carnal, but mighty through God to the pulling down of strong holds."* This verse teaches us that our battle is not a natural battle, but a spiritual one. The Bible also teaches us that the battle is not ours, but that *"the battle is the Lord's."* Our job is not to fight the enemy. Our job is to resist him by using God's Word in prayer. And God says we are to *"fight the good fight of faith."* What He is telling us is to trust Him, follow His Word, and do what we are capable of doing. And He will do for us what we are incapable of doing.

I offer this prayer for those who are involved in this fight:

Lord God, I present to You those who are struggling and feel like they are losing the battle. My prayer is that You will renew their strength, give them encouragement and hope, and let them know the fight is not lost. I thank You, Lord, for the release of wisdom and that from this point on they will fight the good fight of faith, knowing who the real enemy is.

You have made each of us more than conquerors, but in many cases, we have been led to feel that we are less than a conqueror. The adversary has used many tactics against us in his attempt to divert us from the right path. Your Word says that if we acknowledge You in all of our ways, You will direct our paths. We receive victory over the enemy. In Jesus' name. Amen.

Chapter 10

GOD'S SUCCESSFUL FORMULA

*"Finally, my brethren, be strong in the Lord,
and in the power of his might." —Ephesians 6:10*

God created us in His image and in His likeness and gave us power and dominion. If your desire is to walk in power, your aspiration is consistent with God's design for your life.

In Ephesians 6:10, God's Word tells us to *"be strong in the Lord,"* not in ourselves. We have tried to be strong in ourselves using human solutions concerning the challenges of being overweight and obese. According to the statistics we have failed.

Well-meaning fat loss experts, doctors, scientists, and personal trainers have tried to defeat this problem. Their solution is self-help, which includes developing quick-fix supplements, creating programs that at best yield short-term results, building gyms with expensive memberships, and writing secular books. The health-and-wellness industry is targeted to become the next trillion-dollar industry. But even after all of our exhausted efforts and all of the money we have spent, the epidemic of being overweight and obese is doubling and tripling. Now it is time to be strong in the Lord and in the power of His might, so He can help us win the battle of the bulge.

In this chapter you will learn, through the example of the lives of the children of Israel, how trusting God and following His successful formula through His Word will help you achieve your fat loss goals and true transformation. We will examine the contrast between the lives of the children of Israel and the lives of the Egyptians concerning nutrition, exercise, and being overweight and obese.

A major part of God's plan is our salvation. If we are healthy and vibrant here on earth, yet not prepared to spend eternity in heaven, God's divine purpose has been lost. By implementing God's Word in our daily lives, we can create a physical and spiritual balance. And balance is one of the keys to life and true transformation.

If you acknowledge God in all your ways, even in losing body fat, His Word promises that He will direct you down the path to success. In order to ensure permanent victory over excess body fat, you must follow God's formula. If you do, you will be successful, not only in fat loss, but in every area of your life.

THE CHILDREN OF ISRAEL

The children of Israel embraced God's successful formula for diet, nutrition, and exercise. They did not understand the principles behind God's stance. They had no idea that His eating plan, as outlined in the Old Testament, would someday be validated by a tremendous amount of science. They simply obeyed His voice and reaped the benefits.

One of the benefits they enjoyed was that they were fruitful. Scripture says, *"They increased, multiplied and filled the land."* They were also noted as being "mighty" (Exodus 1:9). Was this a miraculous phenomenon God performed for His people who had favor in His sight? No. They simply followed God's formula for physical and spiritual success.

The Egyptians were afraid of them because the Israelites were stronger and outnumbered them. They wanted to gain complete control over God's people because they were *"more and mightier."* Exodus 1:8–9 says, *"Now there arose up a new king over Egypt, which knew not Joseph. And he said unto his people, Behold, the people of the children of Israel are more and mightier than we."* Webster's definition of *mightier* is "having or showing great power, or physical and bodily strength." The Hebrew definition of *mightier* is "to be powerful, great in number, to be increased, or to break the back of the enemy."

The children of Israel were *"more and mightier,"* and maintained health and longevity for three reasons: they exercised by being made to work *"with rigor and hard bondage,"* the quality of their nutrition was in accordance with God's standards, and they had a strong commitment to please God by following His Word. And God responded by protecting them and giving them what they needed to fulfill His will for their lives.

DIET AND NUTRITION

History and science have shown dramatic differences between the diets of the early Egyptians and the children of Israel. Through archaeology and the study of ancient agriculture in Egypt, we have discovered that in those days the mud was very fertile due in part to early floods. This allowed farmers to grow large crops of barley and wheat. They also grew lots of vegetables, onions, leeks, garlic, beans, and lentils. These foods were the mainstay for the children of Israel.

The Egyptians, on the other hand, ate more land meat, mainly because they could afford the high cost. One Egyptian delicacy was stuffed door mice. They also enjoyed eating duck, geese, pigeons, pelicans, oxen, gazelle, wild boar, sheep, goat, and antelope.

The children of Israel were poor, so they ate mainly fish and vegetables, which is in accordance with God's dietary laws. They didn't know why God instructed them not to eat certain things, they just obeyed His voice. By following the Word of God, they were blessed and lived longer.

The Egyptians didn't honor God, nor did they follow His dietary laws. In Exodus 5:2, Pharaoh said, *"Who is the LORD, that I should obey his voice to let Israel go? I know not the LORD, neither will I let Israel go."* The Egyptians held God's word in blatant disregard.

The Egyptians ate things that were dangerous to their health, but they had no way of knowing this. The only thing the Egyptians had to gauge what they should or shouldn't eat was by what they could see and using mental reasoning. The Egyptians saw that cows had four legs, two eyes, and a tail; a mouse also had four legs, two eyes, and a tail, but it was smaller and harder to catch. To the Egyptians cows and mice were both good for food. But the mouse was not acceptable food in the sight of God. Since the mouse was hard to come by, only the rich could afford this delicacy and it became a common dish at the king's banquets. In those days, people had no way of tracking the cause of rabies, or other deadly diseases, that came from ingesting what they considered to be food. The Egyptians contracted parasites that weakened their immune systems. They died of parasitic diseases and viruses caused by what they ate.

God protected His people with love, by instructing them not to eat what would cause harm and possibly death. It wasn't necessary for the children of Israel to understand the science of why God said not to eat these things. They simply looked up to a loving Father and trusted that He had their best interest at heart.

The children of Israel followed God's dietary laws; as a result, they were protected from disease. They ate in a way that made them healthier than their taskmasters, the Egyptians. God protected them from anything that was inconsistent with building and strengthening their bodies by excluding those substances from their food regimen. Their immune systems had the proper nutrients to maintain optimal health. If any type of virus or disease attacked them, their bodies could fight it off. No wonder the children of Israel lived longer, had fewer stillborn babies, and had less disease claiming their lives.

We have discussed the positive and negative effects of what was eaten by the children of Israel and the Egyptians in biblical days. It was very important for the children of Israel to obey God regarding what they ate. In their day and age they didn't have access to the knowledge we have today concerning food. The Bible clearly states that in the last day's knowledge would increase {Daniel 12:4}. It is important for us to use the knowledge that God has given us through His Word, which fits perfectly with true science. This will maximize our health, including the reduction of body fat.

FOOD VERSUS POISON

Most of us consider food to be what we eat, but is this truly the definition of food? *Food* is actually defined as any nourishing substance eaten, drunk, or otherwise taken into the body to sustain life, provide energy, and promote growth and health. In Genesis 1:11, we read that God created fruits and vegetables. He also gave us animals for meat {Leviticus 11}. These foods contain all the vital nutrients we need to live a healthy balanced life.

Poison is defined as a substance that has an inherent tendency to destroy life or impair health. Ask yourself if what you put in your mouth more closely resembles the definition of food or poison. If we are completely honest, most of us would have to admit that a considerable amount of what we eat is more similar to poison rather than what God regards as food. Many of the things we eat are not life sustaining, do not provide nourishment or promote health, but actually impair health and can cause cancer, obesity, and eventually death. Oftentimes the things we eat include dangerous chemicals known as carcinogens, and are so processed and stripped of nutrients they no longer contain life-enhancing properties.

We have developed a taste for high-glycemic, highly processed, carcinogenic types of food. These foods satisfy our newly evolved taste buds, cravings, and addictions, but they yield empty calories that contribute to being overweight and obese.

Today, we are losing the battle of being overweight because we have accepted the concepts of the Egyptians, such as self indulgence, self-will, our own intellect, and following human solutions for fat loss. We are trying to be effective against a problem that can only be resolved through God's power. It would be wise to avoid the practices of the Egyptians, who ate things that were hazardous to their health.

Most Christians pray before meals. We ask God to bless our food, even when we know that what we are eating or drinking is counter-productive to the advancement of our health and longevity. Instead of praying and asking God to bless what we know to be harmful to our health, why not take a different approach by asking God to help us change our bad habits concerning what we eat?

FORCED EXERCISE

The Egyptians felt threatened by the children of Israel and decided something must be done to weaken this people who posed a threat to their kingdom. They decided to work God's people to death, literally. But the more they worked the children of Israel, the more they multiplied; the heavier the burden, the stronger they became {Exodus 1:11-13}. As the Egyptians increased the workload (exercise), God's people became stronger. The Bible says they "*afflicted them*" {Exodus 1:12}. The affliction and the rigor that they endured was a major increase in their workload.

The Egyptians did not understand that when you increase exercise and eat properly it only serves the purpose of making you stronger, building your immune system, and giving you more endurance. The attempt of the Egyptians to weaken God's people only contributed to making them stronger. This is a perfect example of the benefits of bodily exercise.

In 1 Timothy 4:8, the Bible tells us, "*Bodily exercise profiteth little: but godliness is profitable unto all things.*" Some well-meaning Christians have taken this scripture and misconstrued it by saying it's not important to participate in physical exercise. Let's expound on the meaning of this passage.

The intention of this text is to point out that though physical exercise profits us while we are here on earth, godly exercise will profit us throughout eternity. When we leave this earth we will put on a glorified body. There will be no use for this vessel made of clay. It will go back to the dust from which it came. We will not need physical exercise as we know it now.

Some have used this Scripture as an excuse not to exercise. This type of thinking has contributed to the increase of excess body fat. God never intended for this passage to be used as an excuse. Our bodies are the temples God wants to dwell in, and we should give Him a house that performs at the highest level possible. Being unhealthy from lack of exercise and poor nutrition is not a threat to your salvation; it does not mean you won't make it to heaven. As a matter of fact, your unhealthy state just might cause you to get to heaven a little faster.

OUR COMMON ENEMY

The Egyptians failed in their attempts to destroy the children of Israel. This notable fact was disturbing to the Egyptians, so they devised a different strategy to diminish the Israelites. They sent midwives to the Hebrew women. When the mothers were delivering their children, the midwives were ordered to kill every male child and allow only the female children to live. In Exodus 1:15–16 the Bible states, *"The king of Egypt spake to the Hebrew midwives, of which the name of the one was Shiphrah, and the name of the other Puah: And he said, When ye do the office of a midwife to the Hebrew women, and see them upon the stools; if it be a son, then ye shall kill him: but if it be a daughter, then she shall live."*

This attempt to kill the baby boys didn't work. So, the Egyptians made another attempt to destroy God's people by casting the baby boys into the river to drown with the intention of preventing Moses, the deliverer, from setting God's people free. God preserved His life because the children of Israel had put their trust in Him. God saw the children of Israel being afflicted and mistreated, so it was only a matter of time before God stepped in to vindicate His people. In Psalms 34:19 the word of God says, *"Many are the afflictions of the righteous: but the Lord delivereth him out of them all."*

The Egyptians couldn't do anything to stop God's people from increasing in number by being healthy and living longer with a better quality of life.

God's people today have an enemy, too. Satan wants to destroy us. John 10:10 says, *"The thief cometh not, but for to steal, and to kill, and to destroy."* But, if we follow God's direction like the children of Israel did, our enemy's desire to diminish us by making us overweight or obese, or by shortening our lives, will be ineffective.

If the enemy fails in his quest to destroy you, he will try to make your life miserable by stealing your joy, causing depression, and making you discontented with who you are and how you look. This is his job and he is very good at it.

The epidemic of being overweight and obese is a powerful tool the adversary is using to defeat God's people by causing us to be ineffective, depressed, without energy, sick, diseased, and ultimately to die early deaths.

Natural Laws and Spiritual Laws

God wants us to realize that we have more power and are stronger than we think we are, but power unrealized is power unused. The Lord wants us to raise our level of thinking to a new plane, or paradigm. All the benefits He has for us are written in Scripture. These are not just promises; they are spiritual laws.

Most of us are a lot more familiar with natural laws than spiritual laws. So it's easier for us to believe the natural laws. For example, when you put water in the freezer overnight, you don't pray it will become ice. You don't stay up all night coaching the water to get cold and freeze. If the temperature is low enough the water will freeze. Another example: if you plant a seed, you don't worry about it growing downward and the roots growing out of the ground. That would be contrary to the laws of nature, which causes plants to grow toward the sun.

If we can believe this, why do we struggle with spiritual laws? God made the natural laws as well as the spiritual laws. If we allow Him to direct us, as we submit to these natural and spiritual laws, we will see a positive change in our physical and spiritual bodies.

God often speaks in parables to help us understand spiritual concepts by comparing them to natural events that we can easily relate to; such as rain falling from the sky. Rain serves several objectives, including contributing to plant growth, nourishing human and animal life, and replenishing the earth's bodies of water. When God decides rain is necessary, the rain accomplishes what it was sent to do. It does not evaporate and return to the clouds until His desire has been accomplished. This is a natural law.

Even more powerful, God sent His Word to the earth, like the rain, and it will not return to Him without accomplishing what it was sent to do. Isaiah 55:10–11 says:

For as the rain cometh down, and the snow from heaven, and returneth not thither, but watereth the earth, and maketh it bring forth and bud, that it may give seed to the sower, and bread to the eater: So shall my word be that goeth

forth out of my mouth: it shall not return unto me void, but it shall accomplish
that which I please, and it shall prosper in the thing whereto I sent it.

As God's people, we need to find out what His Word has to say about our health, which includes the excess body fat we are carrying. Hebrews 12:1 says, *"Lay aside every weight, and the sin which doth so easily beset us, and let us run with patience the race that is set before us."* There is a spiritual and physical parallel here. If you hold onto excess spiritual weight, it will hinder your spiritual health. The Bible says, lay it aside. By the same token, if you hold on to excess physical weight, it will hinder your physical health. God wants you to lay this aside too. If you are struggling with diet and nutrition, it is time to allow God to take out the struggle.

ASK AND YOU WILL RECEIVE

The Egyptians followed their own way. They were powered by their own strength and might, using human intellect, natural reasoning, and self-will. As we have seen, this path leads to failure.

If you desire to follow God's Successful Formula for your life; including, the development of godly habits concerning diet and exercise then pray this prayer with a sincere heart, believing that God answers prayer:

Lord, I bow my heart to ask for Your help. Your Word tells me I have not because I ask not. So I am asking You to help me think, feel, and act differently concerning what I put in my mouth. I ask You to give me the discipline and the ability required to overcome being overweight. All of my efforts have failed because I have lacked the most important ingredient: I have not acknowledged You to the degree I should have in this area of my life. I ask You to forgive me for not including You, for not seeking Your guidance for the answer to a problem only You can rectify.

I have struggled with being overweight and it has hindered me in becoming all You want me to be. I read in Your Word that I am "more and mightier," but at times I feel "less and weaker." So God, I commit to You to change what I have done in the past, realizing this can't be done without Your successful formula. I confess that I can do all things through Christ, who is my strength. Thank You, Lord. In Jesus' name. Amen.

God has not changed. As He gave the children of Israel what they needed, He will also give you what you need. Do you need more will-power? God will supply it. Do you require discipline? God will supply it.

Man does not have the answer. The only real solution is going back to the basics and getting back to God's Successful Formula. By doing this you will succeed in every area of your life, including permanent fat loss and true transformation.

Fat Loss for Life
(*The Plan*)

Chapter 11

THE POWER OF 21

"Beloved, I wish above all things that thou may prosper and be in health, even as thy soul prospers." —3 John 1:2

It is scientifically proven that it takes twenty-one days of consistent activity to change an already developed habit. It also takes twenty-one days of consistent activity to create a new habit.

A habit is an action or a series of actions performed subconsciously. Your subconscious mind records every word, feeling, and action that has taken place. These events are stored, and used later, to create patterns of how you view and act in similar situations as they occur throughout your life. For instance, if every time a child falls down or gets hurt her mother attempts to soothe her by giving her ice cream, as she grows she most likely will associate eating something sweet with comfort. Her subconscious association will lead to a habit of eating pleasure foods in painful or stressful situations, which typically contributes to the increase of excess body fat.

It is important you don't mistake formed habits for spiritual addictions – they are distinctly different. An addiction is a counter-productive relationship with something you have become dependent on, which must be dealt with spiritually. A habit is something you have repetitively done and subconsciously it has become natural for you to do. Regardless, if you are dealing with a habit or an addiction, nothing is too hard for God. The objective of "The Power of 21" is to keep good habits, and to replace bad habits with new ones that are conducive for reaching your physical and spiritual goals.

If you consistently perform a new action for twenty-one days, the new action will form a behavioral pattern that becomes more natural for you. Even four days of consistently performing a new action is beneficial because it encourages you to believe that the new action is something you can accomplish. As more time passes, you feel more confident and comfortable with the new behavior. Each day of success multiplies upon the previous day's success, giving you a sense of achievement. The longer you consistently repeat the newly adapted behavior, the more permanent it becomes. After you continuously perform the new behavior for twenty-one days, your subconscious mind automatically engages in the newly adopted behavior. You will find what used to be hard-to-impossible to perform requires less effort, since you have now developed a new habit.

A biblical record of one of God's servants using the principle of "The Power of 21" is in Daniel 10. Daniel set his face toward God to seek understanding and, at the same time, he consecrated himself to God and physically disciplined himself in what he ate for twenty-one days. Daniel received a life changing answer when he applied twenty-one days of seeking God; along with consecutively controlling what he ate. The Word of God lets us know he ate "no pleasant thing." This means he only ate what was essential to sustain his health and countenance.

Daniel gave us a great example of "The Power of 21" by committing twenty-one days to God spiritually, mentally, and physically.

The Faith & Fat Loss Program is designed to lead you to God for producing a life transformation. We are limited when we simply make a change, which means we have the ability to go back to our old habits; but through God's supernatural ability, transformation takes place.

The first phase of the Faith & Fat Loss program is a twenty-one-day jump start based upon biblical principles, consisting of **proper eating**, **Scripture**, **exercise**, and **prayer**. As you consecrate these four areas of your life to God you will develop new habits to assist you in overcoming the battle of being overweight and obese, physically and spiritually.

For twenty-one days you **eat proper** foods that are healthy, balanced and conducive for life, longevity, and fat loss. You study **Scripture** to detoxify your spiritual body and develop new spiritual eating habits. You **exercise** to release natural endorphins, increase energy, and decrease body fat. You **pray** for the Holy Spirit to be your comforter, a deeper relationship with God, and strength to finish the transformation process.

"The Power of 21" is powerful in the fact that when you begin to apply this principle, physically and spiritually, significant changes take place in a short period of time. The first twenty-one days of the Faith and Fat Loss Program is the beginning of your new permanent lifestyle. The habits you develop during the first twenty-one days prepares your physical body to respond to diet and exercise; and prepares your spiritual body to respond to the transforming power of the Word of God and prayer. "The Power of 21" helps you bring your physical and spiritual systems into a healthy and pliable state.

A mistake that many have made after the first twenty-one days is to allow themselves to become lax, as if transformation were complete. You must realize that some of your habits have been developed over many years. They are stubborn and would like to overtake the newly developed habits. So, it is important to maintain the new behaviors. Applying "The Power of 21" in nutrition, Word study, exercise, and prayer not only solidifies your desire for a new lifestyle, but provides an atmosphere for God to transform your life. Once God has done His part there is no going back.

Chapter 12

21-Day Jump Start:

Phase One

"Consecrate yourselves today to the Lord…that He may bestow upon you a blessing this day." —Exodus 32:29

Faith & Fat Loss is designed in two phases to help you best attain your health and fat loss goals. The first phase is a 21-Day Jump Start based on the principles of the "Power of 21." During the initial three weeks you're preparing the way for God to work in your life. Based on this solid foundation, He can take you to new heights of spiritual and physical transformation. The second phase is the lifestyle change designed to continue fat loss until your goals are reached, and is explained and laid out in detail in chapter 13. After you have reached your desired goals, this phase is used to maintain your success for life.

The Faith & Fat Loss 21-Day Jump Start is not a quick fix to weight loss. It is designed to detoxify your fat cells, decrease body fat, and create significant physical and spiritual changes in a short time. And it's only the beginning of the Faith & Fat Loss Program that will lead to a healthier you. This is a complete lifestyle consisting of nutrition, supplementation, exercise, Scripture, and prayer.

In just twenty-one days, you can experience dramatic fat loss. But seeing the numbers on the scale decrease is only one benefit of following this plan. The jump-start also prepares your body to respond to diet and exercise; and your spirit to respond to the transforming power of God's Word and prayer.

CONSECRATION

The 21-Day Jump Start is more than just a new diet to try out. This first twenty-one days is a serious commitment. A consecration.

The definition of *consecrate* is to set aside a period of time to completely dedicate oneself to God—physically, spiritually, mentally, and emotionally.

During this time, all of your actions are committed to God: what you put in your mouth, your physical exercise, the study of Scripture, and prayer. Doing this will empower you to complete the task. When you consecrate yourself to God, you are placing yourself in the best position possible to obtain the permanent fat loss and true transformation you have been longing for.

I praise God for your commitment to this consecration. This is my prayer for your success.

Lord God, I pray for the readers of this book as they embrace this consecration, that they would be strengthened in the power of Your might. That all of the failures they have encountered in the past would work together for their good. I pray that You would take each failure and make it a stepping-stone to draw them closer to You and their success. Lord, allow them to realize that they can do nothing without You. Their success is in Your hands. I thank You that Your desire is for them to be more, and not less; to go up, and not down. Just like with the children of Israel, You want to bring them in and not keep them out. Let them know that they are in the right place, at the right time, as they embrace this consecration, which includes the 21-Day Jump Start that will ultimately result in their victory over excess body fat and the completion of transformation. In Jesus' name. Amen.

WHY JUMP START?

The first twenty-one days of the Faith & Fat Loss program isn't necessarily designed for fat loss, although a tremendous amount of fat loss occurs. The purpose is to build a foundation for permanent fat loss. During this period you will begin the process of detoxifying and building your physical and spiritual body, speeding up the metabolism, and preparing the body for maximum fat loss.

Today's environment is saturated with chemicals and toxins that accumulate and are stored in the body's fat cells. These toxins resist any effort (exercise and diet) to decrease body fat. Our objective is for you to eat specific foods, drink the appropriate type of water, and take the necessary supplements to unlock and open the fat cells, so that the toxins along with the fat can be released. The degree the fat cell is opened determines the amount of fat loss resistant toxins and cellular fat that is released from the cell. If you follow the 21-Day Jump Start closely you will maximize your results, not only in phase one, but it will also assist you in maximizing your results in phase two because the cell has opened as much as it is capable of, giving space to release the fat loss resistant toxins and the extra body fat. If you follow the plan slightly you will receive minimal results because the fat cell will only open slightly releasing a minimal amount of toxins. This will not only affect your results during the first twenty-one days, but it will affect the second phase as well making fat loss slower and more difficult to achieve. The range of fat loss in the first twenty-one days is seven to twenty-seven pounds; how faithfully you adhere to this plan will determine if you will be closer to the seven or the twenty-seven pounds. The amazing thing about the tremendous amount of fat loss is that you are never allowed to be hungry.

With fat loss we must always consider the metabolism. It is safe to say if you carry an excessive amount of body fat your metabolism is suffering. During the 21-Day Jump Start, our goal is to create a healthy metabolism, and a by-product of a healthy metabolism is fat loss.

This twenty-one day period is also a time for detoxifying the spiritual body. We have toxic thoughts and thought processes that have been created through past experiences and circumstances. Detoxification comes through placing yourself in God's presence, studying His Word, and prayer.

SIMPLE RULES

There are a few simple rules (or fat loss principles) that must be followed during the 21-Day Jump Start that will maximize your results. You will find detailed explanations of how and why these rules are so critical to your overall success in the following chapters.

- **The #1 rule is to never eat a carbohydrate alone.** During each meal you must eat a combination of proteins, essential fatty acids, and carbohydrates.
- Never allow yourself to be hungry.
- Eat five to six small meals per day.
- Eat carbohydrates in the proper order. Starchy carbs (complex carbs) should be eaten with the first four meals of the day. Simple carbs should not be eaten during this phase. One of the only exceptions to this rule is the grapefruit and grapefruit juice. Because of the grapefruits defatting and detoxifying properties they can be eaten during any of the first four meals. The grapefruit juice can only be consumed in conjunction with the Ron Williams Food Complex. Fibrous carbs can be eaten during any meal throughout the day. But for the last two meals they are the only carbohydrates allowed.
- Stop eating two hours prior to bed. The only exception is if you experience hunger during this time period; the higher rule of fat loss is never allow yourself to be hungry. So if you are hungry before bed, eat a small amount of protein and an essential fatty acid to hold you over for the night.
- Daily, drink a minimum of 64 oz. of distilled water fortified with approximately 30 drops of Ionic Trace Minerals.
- Every other day do 15-20 minutes of fat burning cardio, at your personal training heart rate. (See chapter 15)
- On the alternate days of the fat burning cardio, do 30 minutes of the Ron Williams IsoDynamic Fat Loss Training, per the guidelines outlined in chapter 15.

- Spend a minimum of 15 minutes per day studying the memorization Scriptures in chapter 14: Food for Life (God's Word.)
- Spend a minimum of 15 minutes praying concerning your fat loss success and spiritual growth. Practice using the Scripture memorization verses in prayer.

Warning: As the chemicals and toxins are being expelled from the body, don't be alarmed if you experience flu-like symptoms and a lack of energy. This is normal with any effective detoxification. A body that is filled with excitotoxins, halogens, and other poisons is resistant to fat loss. It is not abnormal for the body to accumulate 30 lbs. (or more) of these toxic substances.

SIMPLE STEPS

Step 1 – Before starting the 21 Day-Jump Start it's important to record your measurements and weight in the chart found in the exhibits in the back of the book. You will also take the first of a series of pictures to document your on-going success. In chapter 18 you will find detailed instructions on how and when to take your measurements and photos.

Step 2 – One of the most important things in this program is that you are developing a new lifestyle. With this in mind, review the food list below and create a grocery list of foods that will be enjoyable to you during the first twenty-one days. This period will aid you in establishing new habits for your new permanent lifestyle.

Step 3 – Preparation is essential for your success. At the beginning of each week make a plan, according to the foods you have chosen and purchased, of what you will eat and the times you will eat each meal throughout the week. (Remember: Never eat a carbohydrate alone, you must eat it in combination.)

Step 4 – Determine the best time for your daily exercise, prayer, and Word study. Then set a schedule in writing for these activities. You will find a prayer and Word study chart in the exhibit section in the back of the book. In Chapter 15 you will learn some guidelines for establishing a daily exercise routine.

Step 5 – In the tools section at the back of the book you will find a 21 Day success journal. In the journal write your goals, successes, struggles, feelings, physical progress, spiritual progress, and prayers. It is also a place where you can plan your daily meals, exercises, Word study, and prayer time.

Step 6 – Completely consecrate the 21-Day Jump Start period to the Lord in what you eat, your exercise, your prayer life, and your Word study. By consecrating yourself you are doing what you are capable of doing, and you can expect God to do what you are incapable of doing.

Below you will find a comprehensive outline of the Faith & Fat Loss 21-Day Jump Start eating plan:

Food List for Phase One

Protein (one serving with each meal):

All white fish	Beef – extra lean (90-98%)
Chicken breast	Egg whites (whole egg if free range)
Ground turkey	Ron Williams Food Complex
Salmon	Soybeans
Tuna	Turkey breast
Turkey thighs	

Essential Fatty Acids (one serving with each meal):

Avocados	Black currant oil
Borage oil	Flax seeds
Flax seed oil	Raw almonds
Raw almond butter	Salmon
Wheat germ oil (best source)	White Fish

Permissible, but not the best source of EFA: Olive oil

Carbohydrates (one serving with the first 5 or 6 meals):

Simple Carbohydrates (breakfast, morning snack, lunch, and afternoon snack, only):

Not permissible during the first 21 days with the following exceptions:

1.) Grapefruit can be eaten with breakfast or morning snack along with the starchy carbohydrate (grapefruit aids in detoxifying the fat cells).

2.) The Ron Williams Food Complex will aid you in detoxifying the body and decreasing body fat. With this product you can use 100% grapefruit juice (not cocktail), or you can use 2 Tbsp. of organic sugar from beets or cane, and 1 Tbsp. of 100% cocoa.

Starchy Carbohydrates (breakfast, morning snack, lunch, and afternoon snack, only):

All bran	Barley
Black beans	Brown rice
Buckwheat	Chickpeas (garbanzo beans)
Grits	Kidney beans
Lentils	Oat flour
Oatmeal	Red beans
Spinach pasta	Sweet potatoes
White beans	Whole wheat bread(s)
Whole wheat pasta	

Fibrous Carbohydrates (Allowed in all meals, but the only type of carbohydrate allowed for dinner and evening snack):

Asparagus	Bean sprouts
Broccoli	Cabbage
Cauliflower	Celery
Cucumber	Eggplant
Green beans	Green, red, & yellow peppers
Kale	Leeks
Lettuce	Onions
Radishes	Scallions
Shallots	Spinach
Squash	Zucchini

Herbs and Spices:

Allspice	Basil
Cinnamon	Dill
Frank's Hot Sauce	Garlic
Ginger	Lemon
Lime	Mustard (yellow or brown)
Onion powder	Oregano
Paprika	Pepper
Rosemary	Sage
Sea Salt with iodine	Thyme
Vinegar	

Note: It is important to drink a minimum of 64 oz. of distilled water with 30 drops of the ionic trace mineral supplement added to the water. An additional beverage suggestion is caffeine free herbal tea. It is imperative while detoxifying to drink a good source of water. Increasing your consumption of water will assist in detoxifying the body. Replace your soda, fruit juice, coffee, and tea with a good source of water.

This list is not all inclusive. You can substitute other foods not found on this list as long as they have the same nutritional values.

FOODS TO AVOID DURING PHASE ONE

The foods on the phase-one list are essential in decreasing body fat, speeding up the metabolism, and detoxifying the body. Toxins in unhealthy foods gravitate toward fatty tissue and are stored there making the body toxic and fat loss resistant. Stay away from foods that are high in simple or refined sugars, since they are easily converted into body fat.

Following is a partial list of foods to stay away from during the 21 Day Jump Start. Anything comparable to the listed items should also be avoided.

Breads (except whole wheat)	All dairy products
Bagels	Ketchup
White rice	Mayonnaise
Canned foods (if possible)	Butter or butter substitutes
Processed or boxed foods	Jams, jellies, or preserves
Boxed cereals	Ice cream
Potatoes, french fries, chips	Chocolate
Carrots	Candies or cookies
Peas	Fried foods
Corn	Spray cooking oil
Beets	Soda (regular and diet)
Fruit	Beer and alcohol
Honey	Coffee and caffeinated tea
Sugar	Caffeine
Margarine or shortening	Vegetable oils

MSG or MSG derivatives (see exhibit 1 in the back of the book)
Artificial sweeteners (e.g., aspartame, sucralose, saccharin)

Meal Plan: Example One

Breakfast: Scrambled egg whites (or whole eggs if cage free)
Oatmeal (not instant)
Grapefruit
1 tsp. wheat germ oil

Midmorning snack: 8 oz. Ron Williams Food Complex Chocolate Shake

Lunch: Salad with turkey and vegetables, dressing with 1 tsp. wheat germ oil, 1/8 c. apple cider vinegar & spices
Black beans

Afternoon snack: Hard-boiled eggs (cage free)
Sweet potato
1 T. flax seeds (ground or whole)

Dinner: Grilled or baked fish (salmon, snapper, halibut)
Seasoned vegetables (green beans, broccoli, cauliflower, or squash)
Salad, dressing with 1 tsp. wheat germ oil, 1/8 c. apple-cider vinegar & spiced to taste

Evening snack: Sliced turkey breast
¼ medium avocado

As you can see, in each meal we have chosen a protein, an essential fatty acid, and a carbohydrate.

MEAL PLAN: EXAMPLE TWO

Breakfast: Omelet (cage free eggs) with green peppers and onions
Whole-wheat bread, toasted, with 1 tsp. wheat germ oil

Midmorning snack: Hard-boiled eggs (cage free)
12 raw almonds
Raw vegetables (celery, broccoli)

Lunch: Tuna
Fresh green salad with vegetables and avocado
Whole-wheat bread
1/8 c. apple-cider vinegar

Afternoon snack: 8 oz. Ron Williams Food Complex Grapefruit Shake
Sliced chicken breast

Dinner: Grilled chicken breast
Steamed vegetables (asparagus or squash)
Salad, dressing with 1 tsp. wheat germ oil, 1/8 c. apple-cider vinegar and spices

Evening snack: Sliced turkey breast
Small salad, with vinegar and wheat germ oil dressing

21 DAY JUMP START

Daily Food Chart *(Example of eating in combinations)*

	Breakfast	Snack	Lunch	Snack	Dinner	Snack
Protein	Scrambled Eggs (Cage Free)	8 oz. Protein Drink	Tuna Fish Packed in Water	8 oz. Protein Drink	6-8 oz. Grilled Chicken Breast	3-4 oz. Turkey Breast
Essential Fatty Acid	1 tsp. Wheat Germ Oi	12 Raw Almonds	Avocado	1 Tbsp. Ground Flax	Dressing: Wheat Germ Oil & Vinegar	1 tsp. Wheat Germ Oil
Fibrous Carbs.		8 oz. Raw Vegetables			Steamed Veggies & Green Salad	
Starchy Carbs.	Oatmeal (Not instant)		2 Slices of Toasted Wheat Bread	Baked Sweet Potato	Not allowed after 3 p.m.	Not allowed after 3 p.m.
Simple Carbs.	Not allowed during the 21 Day Jump Start!					

During the last two meals don't eat any carbohydrates except fibrous carbohydrates. Make sure you eat your last meal a minimum of two hours before bed.

**To prepare your personal daily food chart, see Exhibit 3
in the back of the book.**

Food Preparation

During the 21-Day Jump Start eat fresh foods, instead of frozen foods; frozen foods, instead of canned. All food should be grilled, baked, boiled, broiled, barbequed, steamed, or prepared in a greaseless pan. The best way to cook many of your foods, including scrambled eggs, meat, or food that is normally fried is in a quarter-cup of water instead of oil, butter, or margarine.

When preparing meals, the first item to consider is your protein source. The second item to consider is the source of the essential fatty acid (EFA). The EFA's, if your desire is to decrease body fat, must be eaten with each meal (you can refer to the food list for good sources of EFA's.) The third food category should be a quality source of carbohydrate. The reason for this order is because it's very easy to obtain carbohydrates through fast food restaurants, vending machines, filling stations, grocery stores, and so on. Good sources of protein and essential fatty acids are not as easy to come by.

Our goal is not only to look healthy on the outside, but
to be healthy on the inside!

REMINDERS FOR YOUR SUCCESS

1. No simple sugars (exceptions are listed on the food list).
2. Don't eat sugar substitutes.
3. Never eat a carbohydrate alone.
4. Don't allow yourself to become hungry.
5. Stop eating two hours before going to bed.
6. Keep healthy snacks on hand at all times.
7. Drink at least 64 ounces of water per day.
8. Exercise for fat loss, not fitness.
9. Eat at least five to six balanced meals per day.
10. Plan your meals ahead.
11. Be consistent.
12. Set realistic goals.
13. Get the family involved by teaching them the principles you've learned. This will help you build a support system.
14. When eating out, choose restaurants that serve the types of foods on the 21-Day Jump Start.
15. After meal four, don't eat complex carbohydrates (such as oatmeal, bread, beans, or potatoes).
16. The most important element for your success is prayer.
17. Study the scriptures concerning comfort, discipline, encouragement, faith, strength, and healing found in the Food for Life – God's Word chapter.
18. Commit and consecrate your eating to God.
19. Visit our Website at www.faithandfatloss.com.
20. Enjoy the process!!

COMMIT TO THE CONSECRATION

Consecration is completely committing and setting yourself aside for God's use. One of the things that made the apostles and prophets of old so successful is that they consecrated their lives to God. They realized that making the commitment of consecration wasn't just for their benefit. Ultimately they were doing it to please God, and they didn't want to let Him down. They reaped benefits from their consecration. You will too if you have the same heart during this life-transforming 21-Day Jump Start.

It is important to understand that this consecration is not just a commitment, but it is commitment plus consecration to God. This means you are not just making a decision to do something that only involves self. You are committing four areas of your life to God for twenty-one days. You must examine whether you really want to be successful with permanent fat loss and transformation. During this twenty-one days you can expect tests and trials that will come against the commitment and consecration that you have made to God. Your mind must be made-up that family barbecues, birthday parties, outings, holiday events, bouts with depression that usually cause you to binge, etc. will not divert you from being successful. Many people endeavor on a consecration and they neglect to count up the costs – so they fail. I encourage you to count up the cost. If you do you will succeed.

Lord, I pray for each person who is committing to this consecration; who has the desire to decrease body fat, physically and spiritually; and who desires complete transformation. I ask that You would give them the courage, the strength, and the stamina to endure whatever may stand in front of them. Lord, there will be pitfalls, stumbling-blocks, and closed doors for them; but we ask that you would make them bigger than any hindrance that might present itself. They are "more than conquerors" and they can do all things through Christ who is their strength. I thank you that they will overcome their soul wounds as they continue on the road to losing the excess physical body fat and achieving true transformation. I accept the victory right now, in the name of Jesus'. Amen.

Congratulations for making the commitment to God to follow this consecration. Once you have committed from the heart, I would like you to sign below. By signing below, it is a written confirmation of the commitment and decision in your heart to fulfill this consecration.

"I, _____, **commit and consecrate** my physical and spiritual eating; and physical and spiritual exercise to God. **I will** complete the Faith & Fat Loss 21-Day Jump Start program, with God's help."

_____

Your Signature

The Faith & Fat Loss prayer warriors are praying and asking God to strengthen those who are going through the 21-Day Jump Start, as well as those who are struggling with soul wounds and trying to forgive their perpetrators. We pray for all those who desire to decrease body fat and experience spiritual transformation. To enter your personal prayer requests, or to be a part of our prayer team, please visit our Web site at www.faithandfat-loss.com.

Chapter 13

FOOD FOR LIFE:

Phase Two

Now that you have "Jump Started" your life (physically, spiritually, mentally, and emotionally) it is time to begin the continuation and maintenance program. Phase two – Food for Life has been specifically designed to continue fat loss until your goals are reached. After you have reached your goals, this phase can be used to maintain your success for life.

Food for Life takes what you have already learned in the 21-Day Jump Start and combines it with the following easy-to-use continuation plan. Below is a road map to help you continue your long-term progress of increasing lean muscle and decreasing body fat.

DISPELLING THE CALORIE MYTH

One of the biggest obstacles in overcoming excess body fat is dispelling the myth that thermodynamics works in the body. The principle of thermodynamics is energy-in and energy-out. When it comes to the body this simply means calorie-in and calorie-out. This is one of the most confusing and misleading myths to long-term fat loss and by following this principle, rather than good science, permanent fat loss can't be achieved.

Some well-known and educated professionals recommend the concept of calorie-in and calorie-out, but most neglect to take into consideration the body's ability to adapt to adverse circumstances — which is our God given ability to survive. There are too many variables to condense fat loss down to a simple equation of calorie-in and calorie-out. Caloric intake is only one of the many variables to decreasing body fat.

Energy-in and energy-out is a well known scientific principle and it works, just not in the body for long-term fat loss. This principle is only effective in the mechanical world, not with living organisms. The human body is the most complex and well designed organism, which responds to the higher principle of survival. Our many survival mechanisms make the principle of calorie-in and calorie-out completely impossible for permanent fat loss.

Decreasing calories is not the first thing that should be done when your desire is to decrease body fat. The first thing that should be done is to discover the root cause or to answer this question, "Why do I carry excess body fat?" Very seldom do we find individuals who are overweight because they eat six or seven thousand calories per day. This happens in a small percentage of the overweight population. More often than not individuals carry excess body fat because their metabolism has been destroyed from low-calorie diets.

HEALTHY METABOLISM

If you have had previous experience with sporadic exercising, or a history of depriving the body of nutrition with low-calorie diets or yo-yo diets, your primary objective should not be to lose weight, but to develop a healthy metabolism. An unhealthy, slow metabolism is one of the largest factors for increasing body fat.

One of the goals of the Food for Life program is to speed up the slow metabolism. This may result in adding a pound or two in the beginning. Don't be alarmed. Be assured that the increase is not body fat and that the numbers on the scale will drop fairly quickly. The pound or two that you put on in the beginning should be viewed as a good investment in your fat-loss program. As a result of your investment, the fat will come off much faster and easier in the near future.

Your metabolism is like a fire. Once you get it started, it requires fuel to keep it going. That fuel is food. There are consequences if you allow the fuel in your body to run out. One of the consequences is that your metabolism will slow down causing your body, through the law of self preservation, to learn to live on less fuel. After your metabolism has slowed, if you increase calories at any point-in-time in the future, your body will produce and store fat.

Your metabolism goes up and down according to the signals you send it. You must make sure the signals you are sending are appropriate for the results you desire to achieve. There are several simple principles or signals found in the Food for Life program that when applied will aid in speeding up your metabolism.

FOOD FOR LIFE: KEY PRINCIPLES

Here are some of the objectives that will be accomplished with the Food for Life Eating Plan:

- Maximum fat loss
- Lean muscle increase
- Optimal health
- Energy
- Longevity
- Healthy metabolism
- Sense of well-being

The following key principles are necessary to achieve the above objectives:

Eat Five to Six Meals per Day

Eating six small meals during the day instead of three large ones makes it much easier for the digestive system to digest all of the nutrients and calories. The digestive juices are not compromised and diluted, thus allowing the smaller amounts of food to be more completely broken down. This is necessary for the body to maximize absorption.

Eating five or six small meals per day also helps keep your blood-sugar levels stable. When your blood sugar is stable, the body has no need to secrete enormous amounts of insulin, the fat-storing hormone, into the bloodstream. This decreases the body's tendency to produce more fat from the high insulin levels. If your blood sugar is stable, your body will release more of the hormone glucagon, which is a release hormone. This hormone causes your body to release fat from the fat cells and facilitates it into the muscle to be used as energy.

It is essential that you never allow yourself to be hungry. During times of hunger, the body craves foods that are fattening and counterproductive to your fat-loss goals. Eating six small meals per day will decrease the desire to binge, and will limit the cravings and hunger that come with most conventional fad diets. And most importantly, when the body experiences hunger it sends a signal of starvation. This causes the metabolism to slow down, learning to live on fewer calories.

With the Faith & Fat Loss Food for Life Eating Plan it is mandatory to eat five to six meals a day to help increase your metabolism and reduce body fat.

Eat Proper Combinations

When striving to decrease body fat, proper combinations of food are essential. **Since your desire is to lose body fat, it is important to never eat a carbohydrate alone.** Most people in this country eat a lot of sugar and refined carbohydrates, such as white bread, packaged foods with the guise of low fat, candy, cakes, and cookies. Ingesting a food that is high in carbohydrates causes a spike in your blood-sugar level. To bring your blood-sugar down to a safe level, the pancreas secretes insulin – the fat storage hormone. Insulin coats the glucose molecules and converts them into triglycerides or blood fat. They are then transported into the fat cells and stored as fat.

The only way to avoid this fat-storage process is to stabilize your blood-sugar levels. Three elements can help you accomplish this: protein, essential fatty acids (EFAs), and fiber. When these three nutrients are eaten in combination with carbohydrates, they help decrease body fat. So whenever you eat a carbohydrate, be sure you eat it in combination with a protein and an EFA.

Orange juice, for example, seems like a relatively good choice for fat loss. But orange juice is a high-glycemic carbohydrate that has little fat, fiber, or protein. If you drink it by itself, it will spike your blood-sugar level and most of the calories will be converted into fat, especially if your metabolism is sluggish to begin with. However, if you eat a teaspoon of wheat germ oil and three eggs while drinking your orange juice you will have a proper combination. These foods in combination enter the bloodstream much slower, preventing a spike in the blood-sugar level. This decreases the amount of insulin that is secreted into the bloodstream. **Even though you have eaten more calories, they are better used and will be less likely to be converted into body fat.**

Many popular diet programs suggest that you eliminate starchy or complex carbohydrates and the simple carbohydrates; only allowing the low calorie fibrous carbohydrates. This is counterproductive to increasing your metabolism. Carbohydrates are essential to speed up your metabolism, increase your overall health, give you more energy, and help you maximize and reach your fat-loss goals. But the order in which carbohydrates are eaten during the day is vital.

- Starchy (complex carbohydrates) should be eaten early in the day (for breakfast, morning snack, lunch, or afternoon snack).
- Simple carbohydrates should be eaten in the middle of the day (for morning snack, lunch, and afternoon snack).
- Fibrous carbohydrates are high in nutrition and low in calories. They can be eaten throughout the day, along with the other carbohydrates, but they are the only carbohydrates that can be eaten for dinner or evening snack.

Stop Eating Two Hours Prior to Bed

An easy-to-apply weight loss principle is simply – stop eating two hours before you go to bed. A two-hour period is sufficient time for the majority of the last meal to digest. Your body goes into a state of semi-hibernation while you sleep, so you don't require as much energy. When your body slows down, you need less fuel. Hence, calories eaten right before bed are more easily stored as fat.

If you get hungry within two hours of bedtime, eat a small portion of protein and a small portion of EFAs to sustain you until morning.

Water: God's Way

Water is the simplest, most effective, least expensive aid to decreasing excess body fat.

It is a fact that PURE water is the most essential element to life and at one time it was readily available to every person on the planet. Today, this is not the case; in fact, it is hard to find a good source of drinking water because most of our waters are filled with toxic chemicals and pollutants.

Our bodies are made up of 60 to70% water. If the only water you drink is tap water (which all tap water is filled with toxins and chemicals) then the majority of your body is filled with toxins that can cause you to become sick, overweight, obese, and fat-loss resistant.

Changing from toxic tap water to "pure" water would be the most productive thing you could do to cleanse the fat cells of the fat causing chemicals. In conjunction with implementing the other key principles in this book, your excess body fat would melt away.

All water is not created equal. The best source of water to drink is distilled water fortified with trace minerals. God provided a natural process of distillation through evaporation from the earth and large bodies of water. As God willed, the evaporated water rained down on the earth and collected the necessary minerals for life and longevity. This process has been diminished by the impurities and pollutants in the atmosphere, and the toxins and chemicals on the ground. In addition, the water treatment plants add more chemicals to the water including chlorine and other fat loss resistant chemicals. Today, the God given process of evaporation and rain can be closely reproduced by distillation and adding ionic trace minerals.

If you weigh 185 pounds or more, slowly work up to one gallon a day of Distilled Water fortified with Minerals. If you are less than 185 pounds, drink at least 64 ounces of distilled water fortified with trace minerals per day. If you participate in strenuous exercise, add six to eight ounces of water for every 15 minutes of vigorous activity. Distilled water can be purchased through a local distiller. If you are unable to find a local distiller the next best source is to purchase distilled water from your local grocery stores. You will then add in approximately 30 drops of ionic trace minerals, which can be purchased from well trusted health food stores or through the Faith & Fat Loss website at www.faithandfatloss.com.

Foods that Aid in Fat Loss

There are no "magic pills" that will take away the extra fat. But the following are a few shortcuts that will aid your progress during the second phase:

- Negative foods are carbohydrates that burn more calories than they possess. For instance, one serving of broccoli may contain 100 calories, but requires 150 calories to absorb and digest. This leaves a deficit of 50 calories. Some examples of negative foods are broccoli, celery, spinach, strawberries, apples, and pineapples.
- Sulfuric foods are foods that are high in digestive sulfur. Sulfur helps to detoxify and cleanse the fat cells from toxins that cause our bodies to become fat loss resistant. Some of these foods are very common in our every day diet; such as, grapefruit, grapefruit juice, garlic, onions, cabbage, beets, radishes, and leeks.
- Cruciferous vegetables include broccoli, cauliflower, greens, cabbage, turnips, etc. If eaten slightly steamed they aid in decreasing the negative effects of estrogen.
- Ron Williams Food Complex is a meal replacement that contains a balance of protein, carbohydrates, and essential fatty acids. This product works to increase the metabolism, and will also aid in reversing some of the effects of estrogen dominance, halogens, and other toxins. The Food Complex is a complete meal that can be used as a substitute for any of your daily meals. It can also turn your coffee into a meal by adding two scoops along with either organic honey or sugar.

CONTINUATION & MAINTENANCE PROGRAM

FOOD LIST FOR PHASE TWO

Protein (one serving with each meal):

All white fish	Beef – extra lean (90-98% fat free)
Chicken breast	Egg whites (whole egg if free range)
Goat's milk	Ground turkey
Nonfat cheese	Organic cottage cheese
Organic low-fat dairy products	Organic low-fat milk
Rice milk	Ron Williams Food Complex
Salmon	Soybeans
Tuna	Turkey breast
Turkey thighs	Yogurt

Essential Fatty Acids (one serving with each meal):

Avocados	Black currant oil
Borage oil	Flax seeds
Flax seed oil	Raw almonds
Raw almond butter	Salmon
Wheat germ oil (best source)	White Fish

Permissible, but not the best source of EFA: Olive oil

Note: The oils above are ingested as an essential fat and must not be heated or used for cooking.

Carbohydrates (one serving with each meal):

To intensify weight loss, or for a sluggish metabolism, carbohydrates can be excluded from the last meal of the day.

Starchy Carbohydrates (breakfast, morning snack, lunch, and afternoon snack):

All bran	Barley
Black beans	Brown rice

Buckwheat

Corn

Grits

Lentils

Oat flour

Peas

Shredded wheat

Sweet potatoes

White potatoes

Whole wheat pasta

Chickpeas (garbanzo beans)

Cream of wheat

Kidney beans

Long grain rice

Oatmeal

Red beans

Spinach pasta

White beans

Whole wheat bread(s)

Simple Carbohydrates (morning snack, lunch, and afternoon snack):

Agave nectar

Bananas

Carrots

Grapes

Lemon

Mango

Molasses

Organic Sugar

Pears

Pineapple

Apples

Berries

Grapefruit

Honey

Lime

Melons

Oranges

Papaya

Peaches

Tomatoes

Fibrous Carbohydrates (Allowed in all meals, but the only type of carbohydrate allowed for dinner and evening snack):

Asparagus

Broccoli

Cabbage (red and green)

Celery

Eggplant

Green, red, & yellow peppers

Kale

Lettuce

Radishes

Bean sprouts

Brussels sprouts

Cauliflower

Cucumber

Green beans

Greens

Leeks

Onions

Scallions

Shallots	Spinach
Squash (all types)	Zucchini

Herbs and Spices:

Allspice	Basil
Cinnamon	Dill
Frank's Hot Sauce	Garlic
Ginger	Lemon
Lime	Mustard (yellow or brown)
Onion powder	Oregano
Paprika	Pepper
Rosemary	Sage
Sea Salt with iodine	Tabasco
Thyme	Vinegar

Note: It is important to continue drinking a minimum of 64 oz. of distilled water with 30 drops of ionic trace mineral supplement added to the water. Additional beverage suggestions are black and green tea, herbal teas, and coffee.

This list is not all inclusive. You can substitute other foods not found on this list as long as they have the same nutritional values.

CONTINUATION & MAINTENANCE PROGRAM

FOODS TO AVOID

- White breads, breads with enriched flours (including bagels)
- White rice
- Canned food (as much as possible)
- French fries and chips
- Fried foods
- Margarine or shortening
- Chocolate
- Candies and cookies
- Refined sugars
- High-Fructose Corn Syrup
- Highly processed foods
- Soy sauce or Worcestershire sauce
- Steak sauces that are not organic
- Vegetables oils (such as canola oil and corn oil)
- MSG or MSG derivatives (See Exhibit 1 in the back of the book)
- Artificial sweeteners (such as aspartame, sucralose, saccharin)

MEAL PLAN: EXAMPLE ONE

Breakfast: Shredded Wheat breakfast cereal
with skim milk and 1 tsp. of organic cane sugar
8 oz. Glass of skim milk
1 T. Ground flax seed

Midmorning snack: Low-fat cheese (slices, cubes, or sticks)
Apple or grapes
12 Raw almonds

Lunch: Wheat wrap with turkey, cheese, veggies, and mustard
or vinegar
Brown rice and Black beans
¼ Avocado

Afternoon snack: 8 oz. Ron Williams Food Complex Orange Smoothy

Dinner: Ground-turkey meatloaf
Grilled vegetables
Salad, dressed with 1 tsp. wheat germ oil, 1/8 c. apple
cider vinegar & spices

Evening snack: Lean beef tips
Small salad
1 tsp. Wheat germ oil

CONTINUATION & MAINTENANCE PROGRAM

MEAL PLAN: EXAMPLE TWO

Breakfast: Scrambled eggs, in water
                      Buckwheat pancakes
                      Pure maple syrup with honey
                      1 tsp. Wheat germ oil

Midmorning   Hard-boiled eggs
snack: Strawberries
                      12 Raw almonds

Lunch: Fresh green salad with chicken
                      Corn
                      ¼ Avocado

Afternoon   Cottage Cheese
snack: Apple or peach
                      12 Raw almonds

Dinner: Fajita's: Chicken breast
                      Grilled peppers and onions
                      Fajita seasoning (make sure no MSG)
                      Avocado, lettuce, tomatoes, onion
                      Low fat sour cream

Evening   Sliced deli turkey
snack: 1 tsp. Wheat germ oil
                      Celery sticks

CONTINUATION & MAINTENANCE PROGRAM

DAILY FOOD CHART

	Breakfast	Snack	Lunch	Snack	Dinner	Snack
Protein	Scrambled Eggs in Water	Cheese Sticks	Chicken Breast	Cottage Cheese	Ground Turkey Meatloaf	8 oz. High Quality Protein Drink
Essential Fatty Acid	1 tsp. Wheat Germ Oil	12 Raw Almonds	Avocado	12 Raw Almonds	Dressing: 1 T. Wheat Germ Oil & Vinegar	1 T. Ground Flax Seeds
Fibrous Carbs.			Salad with Vegetables		Grilled Vegetables & Salad	
Starchy Carbs.	Buckwheat Pancakes			Whole Wheat Crackers	Not allowed after 3 p.m.	
Simple Carbs.	Pure Maple Syrup with Honey	Orange			Not allowed after 3 p.m.	

Always carry healthy snacks with you in case the unexpected happens, such as getting caught in traffic, delayed at the airport, stuck at work, etc. Protein shakes, cheese sticks, raw nuts, and fruit are a few good examples. This will help you decrease the chance of eating foods that are counterproductive and contrary to your new lifestyle.

**To prepare your personal daily food chart, see Exhibit 3
in the back of the book.**

Just as in phase one, consecrate your eating regimen to God. Pray for His assistance to help you develop your new habits.

The second phase may be a bit more difficult to stick with because you have more flexibility in your food choices. You'll need to be careful not to slip back into old eating habits; such as, eating the wrong foods at the wrong times, eating less than five or six meals per day, and not eating in proper combination. The following chapters on prayer and Scripture will give you the help, hope, and strength you need to achieve your permanent fat-loss and transformation goals.

Chapter 14

FOOD FOR LIFE:

God's Word

*"And Jesus answered him, saying, It is written, that man shall not live by bread alone, but by every Word of God." —***Luke 4:4**

Our physical food should take second position to our spiritual food. Job 23:12 states, *"I have treasured the words of His mouth more than my necessary food."* Job considered his spiritual food, meaning God's Word, such a high priority that he would be more willing to do without physical food, which sustains his body, than spiritual food, which ensured that his spirit didn't suffer loss. Job refused to jeopardize his spiritual health.

If we don't eat physically, we will become unhealthy and eventually die. If we don't eat spiritually, our fate will be the same. We use Job's testimony as an example of the importance of having spiritual food to build our spiritual body.

As you start on your journey of building and strengthening yourself physically and spiritually, you must realize that just as a baby starts off being nourished, milk is required. The baby's body is not mature enough to digest a steak dinner. In our quest for true transformation, we must start with the foundation, which is represented by the milk of the Word. First Peter 2:2 says, *"As newborn babes, desire the sincere milk of the word, that ye may grow thereby."* A good foundation for spiritual growth starts with the basics: the Word of God and prayer. Growing in these areas is a lifelong process.

When we come to God, we need to be changed and cleansed from our old ways. God designated His Word to cleanse us spiritually. As we prayerfully read and study the Word, God causes a cleansing to take place in our hearts. In Ephesians 5:26, the Bible tells us that God wants to replace our old unclean thoughts by washing our minds with His Word.

It is a well-known fact that changing an old thought requires a new thought. Old negative thought processes are counter-productive to transformation. Some of them are actually toxic; for example, thinking you are destined to be fat, that you are unworthy of success, or that you lack the will-power and discipline to eat correctly for any significant length of time. These negative thoughts are developed out of insecurities and soul wounds.

Spiritual Detoxification

To change your old, toxic thoughts, you need to go through a "spiritual detox." This consists of studying Scripture, verse memorization, and prayer. Spiritual detoxification is similar to physical detoxification in principle. Both cleanse the system of impurities and toxins with the purpose of developing a healthy lifestyle.

We begin this "spiritual detox" with a 21-Day Jump Start. During your first twenty-one days you will build a strong physical and spiritual foundation and will develop newly formed habits that should continue throughout your walk with God.

Here's how the 21 day "spiritual detox" program works. First, make a daily appointment with God. Set a specific time to meet with Him every day for twenty-one days. During your appointments with God:

- Spend a minimum of 15 minutes daily studying the Word and committing to memory the Scriptures written below.
- Memorize one Scripture passage every two days. (Ten memory verses are identified later in this chapter). Write them in a journal or on three-by-five cards to use as flash cards. (Be sure to quote the chapter and verse.) On the twenty-first day, you will review the ten verses you have memorized.

- Read the 10 memorization Scriptures and get an understanding of how they pertain to you regarding your successful transformation and fat loss.
- During your prayer time, be sure to pray the Scriptures that pertain to your current struggles.

Committing the Scripture to memory and studying it will be preparation for your future tests. As adverse situations arise, your responsibility is to use the memory Scriptures and trust God during those times. The core of your success is His Word. For example: if you wake-up and feel depressed, spiritually weak, and have a desire to eat food for comfort — you can no longer respond the way you once did. Remember, your old thought process is considered toxic. Your new thought process must be the Word of God, which are your memorization Scriptures. In this example, you would use an encouragement Scripture, a comfort Scripture, or both.

In Luke 4:4, we read about Jesus responding to a time of testing. He was extremely hungry after fasting for forty days, and the adversary suggested He turn the stones into bread. Jesus quoted Deuteronomy 8:3, saying that *"man does not live by bread alone but by every word that proceeds out of the mouth of God."* God's Word was our Savior's foundation, and quoting it from memory is how He achieved victory.

"Spiritual Detox" Memory Scriptures

During the twenty-one days of "spiritual detox," I can guarantee you will encounter struggles, obstacles, and distractions. But you can overcome these difficult circumstances by using the Word of God. The following 10 Scriptures were prayerfully chosen to help you gain victory in your struggles.

Comfort

The adverse circumstances and situations we experience as we go through life cause us to seek for comfort. This is a common point of attack because we were designed to go to God for our comfort. When we are separated from Him, we substitute true comfort with counterfeits. We often look for comfort in the wrong places, such as alcohol, drugs, sex, power, money, and even food. These so-called comforters lead us away from our goal of transformation and God's purpose for our lives.

When you need comfort, and you're tempted to find that comfort in overeating or other self-destructive behaviors, you can turn to these Scriptures:

Matthew 11:28-30 - *"Come unto Me, all ye that labor and are heavyladen, and I will give you rest. Take my yoke upon you, and learn of me; for I am meek and lowly in heart: and ye shall find rest unto your soul. For my yoke is easy, and my burden is light."*

God understands how hard life's tasks can be. He knows the load you are carrying, and He didn't create you to carry such heavy burdens. The solution He has prepared for you is simple. All He requires is for you to come to Him with the pressures life has presented, and He will give rest to your soul.

1 Peter 5:6-7 - *"Humble yourselves therefore under the mighty hand of God, that He may exalt you in due time: Casting all your care upon Him; for He careth for you."*

Pride says, "The answer is within me." Humility says, "I don't have all the answers." Pride says, "I am completely self-sufficient." Humility says, "I need help." Pride won't allow you to acknowledge that you have needs or ask for assistance. Humility causes you to reach out and up, receiving with open arms what God has, so you can be free.

God can meet our every need, including fat loss. As our Father, God wants to take care of us. He wants us to cast all our cares on Him and allow Him to be God.

If pride has you bound, God can set you free. If pride has forced you away from God, He will draw you near. If pride has made you low, through humility God will exalt you.

John 14:16 - *"And I will pray the Father, and He shall give you another Comforter, that He may abide with you forever."*

Jesus came to be a comfort and a refuge in our time of need. But His earthly ministry was limited because He couldn't be in all places at the same time. Prior to His ascension to heaven, He promised He would send us the true Comforter, who is not limited by time or space. This Comforter is the Holy Ghost. Because He can be in all places at the same time, He is available to each of us always.

DISCIPLINE

Discipline is necessary for a godly life. Where there is no discipline, physical and spiritual growth is limited. But the discipline required for transformation is not generated from the power of man. It comes only through God's power. You can attract God's power by studying His Word and prayer.

Whenever you feel a desire to slip, and you're having trouble following the guidelines you've chosen to follow to achieve your fat-loss goals, you can turn to these Scriptures:

1 Corinthians 9:25-27 - *"All athletes are disciplined in their training. They do it to win a prize that will fade away, but we do it for an eternal prize. So I run with purpose in every step. I am not just shadowboxing. I discipline my body like an athlete, training it to do what it should…"*

Being a good physical athlete requires discipline in eating, exercise, and getting proper sleep. To be a good spiritual athlete also requires discipline in eating (the Word), exercise (communication with God), and resting (trusting in God's promises).

Desire alone is not enough. Actions must be coupled with desire to achieve the physical or spiritual results you want.

ENCOURAGEMENT

At various times in life, we all feel alone, lost, or depressed. The answer isn't in ourselves, our friends, or any other secular avenue. True encouragement comes from seeking God through His Word and developing trust in Him. Whenever you feel discouraged about your progress in achieving your fat-loss goals, rely on these Scriptures:

Romans 8:37 - *"We are more than conquerors through Him that loved us."*

Jesus has already defeated our enemies and given us the victory over all our sins and struggles. Through His sacrifice, we are healed and saved in every area of life. You are *"more than a conqueror,"* even over the extra pounds that in the past have refused to leave. Receive God's promise and walk in your newly discovered victory.

Psalm 27:14 - *"Wait on the Lord: be of good courage, and He shall strengthen thine heart: wait, I say, on the Lord."*

God desires for you to trust Him enough to wait patiently, expecting to receive what He has promised. Sometimes in your waiting, feelings of discouragement and doubt may cross your mind, with thoughts of *Why should God do this for me?*

If whatever you are requesting is part of a well-rounded Christian life, you can expect to receive from God the answer to your prayers. The only thing that stands between you and the fulfillment of your request is time. *"Wait, I say, on the Lord."*

FAITH

A meaningful relationship with God is based on faith. Natural circumstances and the adversary will attack your faith in order to hinder your relationship with God by trying to cause doubt in His Word. When your faith is attacked, trust in the Word. As you do, your faith will grow.

Hebrews 11:6 -*"But without faith it is impossible to please Him: for he that cometh to God must believe that He is, and that He is a rewarder of them that diligently seek Him."*

We cannot please God without having faith. What this means is that if you have faith you have the ability to please God and also that He responds to faith. If your faith is weak, you can exercise to strengthen your faith. The main exercise for building faith is found in Romans 10:17, *"Faith cometh by hearing, and hearing by the word of God."*

STRENGTH

The strength needed for transformation is not generated from the power of man. It is only through God's power and strength. You can attract God's power from studying His Word and being in His presence.

When you are spiritually weak you are vulnerable to the enemy's attacks and without God's strength the risk of failure is high. God desires you to be in His presence because this is where you will experience joy and spiritual strength.

Philippians 4:13 - *"I can do all things through Christ which strengthens me."*

We can do all things pertaining to God and godliness, not with our own strength but with His. We must be strong in the power of the Lord's might. If we wait on the Lord He will renew our strength.

The excess weight you have been carrying, physically and spiritually, has been there far too long. Ask God for the strength to shed that excess weight, and accept the power that He provides for you.

HEALING

God's desire is to heal each of us in every area of our lives. As we draw closer to Him, we will find ourselves being made whole.

If you have a soul wound and you are overweight allow God to heal your hurting soul to begin your lifelong journey of health, fat loss, and transformation.

Psalm 41:4 - *"I said, Lord, be merciful unto me: **heal** my soul…"*

David understood that God wanted to heal him physically, spiritually, and financially, but God's greatest desire was to heal his soul. David's cry unto God was *heal my soul*. David was financially well off, and his relationship with God was constantly growing. But before he could maximize his relationship with God, the pain from his soul wounds had to be healed. He prayed to God for healing of the soul.

You too can ask God to heal your soul.

Exodus 15:26 -*"I am the Lord that healeth thee."*

God is not suggesting that He is our healer. He is making a declaration that cannot be changed. He is saying this is who I AM. If your soul needs to be healed I AM the only one who has the ability to do it. God's desire is for you to bring all of your soul struggles to Him because He said, "*I AM.*" I AM means whatever you need or whatever you are lacking - I AM. In other words, He makes up the difference. What you don't have physically, spiritually, financially, mentally, and emotionally, God will supply.

It is important for every Christian to spend time becoming familiar with God's Word, but the memorization Scriptures above are specifically for the benefit of your transformation and fat loss.

BEYOND THE TWENTY-ONE DAYS

After your "spiritual detox," you will have created a spiritual habit. The continuation of this habit will help you to lay aside every physical and spiritual weight that would hinder the completion of your transformation.

To enhance your memorization of God's Word, add more Scriptures to the ones given above by exploring the Bible and using it as a complete comprehensive study-guide for your success.

Committing to memory God's Word can help increase your prayer life, further your walk with God, and achieve your fat loss goals by:

- Empowering you against the attacks of the enemy.
- Furthering your understanding of His Word.
- Increasing your spiritual maturity.
- Encouraging and strengthening you.
- Bringing you comfort.
- Increasing your faith.
- Helping you to develop discipline.
- Maximizing your ability to achieve transformation.

MY PRAYER FOR YOU

I would like to close this chapter with a prayer for you.

Lord God, Just as we eat physically, we have learned that we must also eat spiritually. Our spiritual body relies on us to take in proper nourishment, which is the Word of God. Lord, help the reader of this book in their quest to build their physical and spiritual body. Help them to develop a healthy spiritual diet. We pray that each Scripture they memorize during this twenty-one day "spiritual detox" would be impactful and effective. We give you praise for the new habits acquired. We commit each one into Your hands and we pray for their spiritual size to increase, as their physical size decreases. In Jesus' name, Amen.

Chapter 15

Exercise:

Fat Loss not Fitness

"Physical training is of some value (useful for a little), but godliness (spiritual training) is useful and of value in everything and in every way, for it holds promise for the present life and also for the life which is to come." —1 Timothy 4:8

In First Timothy 4:8 the Lord is saying two things. The first: physical exercise is valuable. The next: spiritual exercise is more valuable.

A complete and effective fat-loss program must consist of adequate physical and spiritual exercise. Physical exercise is one of the keys to long-term fat loss and health.

As a fat loss expert, a fitness coach, an elite athlete, and a professor of exercise physiology I have learned that there are two very distinct paths that can lead to the loss of body fat. For years, I trained athletes in several different sports to compete on a national and an international level. The fitness principles that were applied increased their performance and made it easier for them to achieve success in the specific sport they were competing in; a secondary bonus of applying these principles was they lost body fat.

For the past twenty-five years, I have personally trained and coached individuals in fitness and fat loss, but approximately ten years ago my focus and heart switched to solely training and helping individuals acquire permanent fat loss. I had seen the frustration and hopelessness that so many people felt from trying again and again, only to fail at their attempts to decrease body fat. So, I designed an exercise program that specifically addresses how to effectively decrease excess body fat through sending proper signals of fat loss, not fitness.

Fitness vs. Fat Loss

There is a distinct difference when it comes to exercising for fitness versus fat loss. You will be happy to learn that there is a difference in fitness exercise and fat loss exercise. Many exercise programs which are prescribed to those who desire to lose body fat have some fat loss principles, but are primarily designed around a fitness activity. This causes these programs to be short-lived and discouraging because they are too difficult and uncomfortable for most individuals to sustain. Fitness exercise is designed around athletic principles, which may end in fat loss. But fitness is not a direct approach to acquiring long-term fat loss, nor is it specifically designed for fat loss.

When your focus is fitness, it requires high performance exercise, which includes high intensity, high impact, duration, and frequency. The difference when you desire fat loss is that the exercise routine is much easier, requires less intensity, is low-impact, and involves less time, but it does require sending a consistent signal.

At right, I have shown an example of twelve principles used by a natural bodybuilder, which includes both fitness and fat loss principles. Although fat loss is achieved, less than 1% of the population desires to follow this strenuous of a program. The bodybuilder's regimen is done to prepare for a competition, not for a permanent lifestyle. When the competition is over, the athlete's body fat will increase. A fitness oriented program has short-term results compared to a fat loss program, which is a lifestyle.

12 Fitness and Fat Loss Principles
for Healthy Natural Bodybuilding

20 minutes of consistent Cardio *** *Fat Loss Principle*	Glycogen Storage Cardio *** *Fitness Principle*	Glycogen replacement meal *** *Fitness Principle*	Never eat a carb alone *** *Fat Loss Principle*
Eat 5 to 6 small meals per day *** *Fat Loss Principle*	Drink 64 ounces of distilled mineral water daily *** *Fat Loss Principle*	Ron Williams IsoDynamic Fat Loss Training *** *Fat Loss Principle*	Eat carbs in proper order *** *Fat Loss Principle*
Resistance Training for muscle mass *** *Fitness Principle*	Chromium *** *Fitness Principle*	Intense Track Leg Training *** *Fat Loss Principle*	Heavy Squat Training *** *Fitness Principle*

Aerobic Kick Boxing is another fitness exercise that is often touted as a fat loss program. This is a high-impact, intense program that applies both fitness and fat loss principles. Again, this makes it very hard for most individuals to participate in because of the high level of fitness required. For example, if you are one-hundred pounds (or even twenty-five pounds) overweight you most likely don't want, as a primary goal, to balance on one leg kicking the other leg into the air rotating continuously from one leg to the other trying to get an aerobic effect. No doubt, this activity is fitness. The side-to-side motion might get you moving, but it does not focus on your primary goal of fat loss.

12 Fitness and Fat Loss Principles of Aero-Kick Boxing

Interval Training	Aerobic Training	Anaerobic Training	Flexibility Training
***	***	***	***
Fitness Principle	*Fat Loss Principle*	*Fitness Principle*	*Fitness Principle*
Footwork and kick training	Glycogen storage training	Coordination and balance	Glycogen storage eating
***	***	***	***
Fitness Principle	*Fitness Principle*	*Fitness Principle*	*Fitness Principle*
Fuel your body to perform	High-impact Training	Advanced exercise	Choreography
***	***	***	***
Fitness Principle	*Fitness Principle*	*Fitness Principle*	*Fat or Fitness Principle*

Even though fitness exercise can benefit your health, and through its strenuous nature may even help in acquiring a limited amount of fat loss, it is not specifically designed for fat loss. Those who are overweight or obese are not interested in fancy footwork, learning how to punch correctly, or spending a lot of time building energy in the muscle, so they can perform on the same level as an athlete.

The body only responds to signals. If you send fitness signals, you will achieve fitness. If you send fat loss signals, you will achieve fat loss. The more fat loss signals you send consistently the faster you will achieve your desired results. Below, we will show you twelve fat loss signals (through eating and exercise) that will produce long-term fat loss.

12 Fat Loss Principles (Signals)

Never eat a carb alone *** *Fat Loss Principle*	Eat carbs in proper order *** *Fat Loss Principle*	Eat 5 to 6 meals per day (Never be hungry) *** *Fat Loss Principle*	Drink 64 ounces of distilled mineral water daily *** *Fat Loss Principle*
Fat-Burning Cardio for 20 minutes *** *Fat Loss Principle*	Ron Williams IsoDynamic Fat Loss Training *** *Fat Loss Principle*	Chromium *** *Fat Loss Principle*	Rid the body of fat loss resistant chemicals *** *Fat Loss Principle*
L-carnitine *** *Fat Loss Principle*	Iodine *** *Fat Loss Principle*	Stress Management & Soul Wound Freedom *** *Fat Loss Principle*	Increased oxygen from Eleuthro *** *Fat Loss Principle*

Fat Loss Exercise Plan

I have created the Faith & Fat Loss exercise program that concentrates solely on fat loss, through a concrete understanding of the differences between fitness and fat loss. With this exercise program I am going to teach you how to work smarter, not harder, and how to finally acquire the permanent fat loss you've been longing for.

Your body responds to repetitive signals, so it is important that you send a consistent signal of fat loss. Prescribed below are six days of exercise that will help you maximize your fat loss goals:

DAY	TYPE of EXERCISE	TIME
Monday	Fat-Burning Cardio	15-20 minutes
Tuesday	IsoDynamic Fat Loss Training	30 minutes
Wednesday	Fat-Burning Cardio	15-20 minutes
Thursday	IsoDynamic Fat Loss Training	30 minutes
Friday	Fat-Burning Cardio	15-20 minutes
Saturday	IsoDynamic Fat Loss Training	30 minutes
Sunday	Day of Rest	

The combination of Fat-Burning Cardio and IsoDynamic Fat Loss Training are the basis of this program, and they are explained in detail in the next section.

TYPES OF EXERCISE

Fat-Burning Cardio

Fat-burning cardiovascular training is exercise specifically focused on training your heart and achieving maximum fat loss; it includes exercises such as walking, jogging, stepping in place, jumping on a miniature trampoline, or jumping jacks. I recommend walking as the best choice for fat-burning cardio because it is the easiest to monitor, it doesn't require any accessories, and can basically be done anywhere.

The way to most effectively burn body fat through cardio is to exercise at your "training heart rate" for a minimum of fifteen minutes, at least three days a week.

Your objective is to reach your training heart rate. The way to accomplish this is to walk with your hands above your heart at a pace that is slightly uncomfortable, but yet you are still able to talk (whichever exercise you choose, the formula is the same.) Starting slightly below your training heart rate is more productive than starting above your training heart rate. There are three reasons you don't want to exercise above your training heart rate:

1. If your intensity is too high, it will cause excess fatigue.
2. By overexerting yourself, your exercise regimen will be less enjoyable, which makes it harder to stay consistent. And without consistency you will not achieve the results you desire.
3. **Exercising above your training heart rate causes you to burn carbohydrates rather than sending a signal to burn fat for the next twenty-four hours.**

We want to reiterate that when it comes to exercise, harder does not mean you will achieve more fat loss – it actually means the opposite. Remember, you are developing a permanent lifestyle rather than a quick fix.

Ron Williams IsoDynamic Fat Loss Training

IsoDynamic Fat Loss training is a type of circuit training. It is a combination of resistance and fat-burning cardiovascular exercise. To achieve long-term healthy fat loss, both components are needed.

IsoDynamic Fat Loss training concentrates on fat loss, muscle strength, and endurance. This combination generates an abundance of oxygen in the body, which increases fat burning while building lean muscle. This combination will shorten the time you spend working out and will enhance your body's fat-burning capacity. IsoDynamic Fat Loss Training with resistance bands is the safest and most effective way to sculpt and shape your body.

On the days that you perform the IsoDynamic Fat Loss Training you will begin your workout with a short warm-up and stretching. Then you will follow with eight exercises starting with the larger muscle groups and then going to the smaller muscle groups. You will finish with a cool-down and stretching. This will take a total of 30 minutes.

Warm-up & Stretching	3 minutes
Squats (buttocks, upper legs)	30 seconds
Cardio	30 seconds
(repeat 3 times)	
Side-Steps (buttocks, hips)	30 seconds
Cardio	30 seconds
(repeat 3 times)	
Calf raises (calves)	30 seconds
Cardio	30 seconds
(repeat 3 times)	
Standing Chest Press (chest)	30 seconds
Cardio	30 seconds
(repeat 3 times)	
Up-right rows (shoulders)	30 seconds
Cardio	30 seconds
(repeat 3 times)	
Overhead Triceps Extensions (back of arms)	30 seconds
Cardio	30 seconds
(repeat 3 times)	
Standing Bent-over Rows (upper back)	30 seconds
Cardio	30 seconds
(repeat 3 times)	
Biceps Curls (front of arms)	30 seconds
Cardio	30 seconds
(repeat 3 times)	
Cool-Down and Stretch	3 minutes

NOTE: You are welcome to extend the warm-up and cool-down.

The way to be successful while doing this type of training is to keep your body moving at a consistent pace maintaining your training heart rate. Advance from the resistance exercise to the cardio exercise (such as, walking in place, jogging in place, step, miniature tramp, aerobic slide, or jumping jacks) within three to five seconds, and from cardio back to the resistance within three to five seconds, so that you maintain your training heart rate. It is more important to stay consistent than to start out like a tornado and fizzle out at the end.

The reason consistency is so important is that during the first three minutes of cardiovascular exercise, your body burns carbohydrates as its primary source of fuel. If you remain constant, the primary source of fuel becomes fat and this sends a signal to the body to burn body fat for the next twenty-four hours. Because your desire is to decrease body fat it is important to maintain the fat loss signal by not resting. If the transition from the resistance to cardio and vice-versa takes longer than five seconds you lose the fat loss training effect.

Parameters to keep your Workout Safe and Effective

Following these basic principles during your workout sessions will help you safely achieve maximum results:

1. Warm-up and stretch properly before each training session.
2. Keep your body moving continuously.
3. Keep your training heart rate consistent.
4. Don't allow yourself to rest between repetitions.
5. Don't allow yourself to rest between sets.
6. Keep muscles tight during the complete range of motion.
7. Exhale during the initial movement of the repetition.
8. Never sacrifice form and technique for increased resistance.
9. When an exercise requires you to stand, make sure your knees are slightly bent — maintaining good posture.
10. With all upper-and-lower-body exercises, keep the muscles of the lower back contracted.
11. Avoid jerky movements, stay consistent and controlled.

WARM-UP, STRETCH, AND COOL DOWN

Warm-Up

The term *warm-up* is very fitting for what is needed prior to stretching and exercise. Muscles, like rubber bands, are more apt to tear when they are cold. A pre-exercise warm-up session will heat the muscles, so they can stretch more easily.

You need to warm-up prior to exercise in order to prevent injury. Sixty percent of all injuries derived from physical training happen within the first ten minutes of exercise.

Stretch

Stretch for a few minutes before you begin your exercise routine to prepare your body for a successful workout. Muscular flexibility is an essential part of overall health and quality of life. Many joint, muscle, and skeletal problems are the result of poor flexibility. Flexibility is important for good posture, and also contributes greatly to preventing injuries. The efficiency, performance, and energy of a muscle is directly related to its flexibility.

You can use the time during stretching to meditate on God helping you through an enjoyable and effective workout. You can also think about using proper form and technique, as you focus on each movement throughout your training session.

Cool-Down

After you complete your workout, cool-down to minimize soreness. The cool-down process will also enhance recovery from your workout.

By embracing the exercise portion of this program you are implementing a vital key to decrease excess body fat, and increase health and longevity. I would like to pray that God would help you enjoy your new lifestyle of exercising consistently and effectively to accomplish your goals for permanent fat loss and transformation.

Lord God,

I thank You for those who have made the decision to make this lifestyle change by implementing the Faith & Fat Loss exercise program. I ask that You would give them the discipline to develop this new lifestyle and that it would become something that they enjoy. I pray that You would give them what it takes to overcome excess body fat, depression, low self-esteem, a lack of energy, and a decreased lifespan. Your Word clearly states that we can do all things through Christ that strengthens us. In order to have Your strength, we also need Your joy because the joy of the Lord is our strength. Let them experience the strength that comes from walking in Your joy. In Jesus' name. Amen.

As a member of our website you will find additional exercises and video footage on how to safely and properly perform the exercises. To learn more visit www.faithandfatloss.com.

Chapter 16

SPIRITUAL EXERCISE:

Prayer

"And ye shall seek me, and find me,
when ye shall search for me with all your heart." —Jeremiah 29:13

The definition of *exercise* is "to exert energy for muscle development." Exercise usually relates to building the physical body, but we also have spiritual muscle that needs development. Physical exercise takes place with the physical body and is more familiar to each of us because it takes place in the natural world of what is seen, touched, and heard. On the other hand, spiritual exercise takes place in the unseen world. **Spiritual exercise is the soul on its knees, before God in prayer.**

Just like there is a parallel between physical exercise and spiritual exercise; there is also a parallel between a physical body and a spiritual body. It is important for Christians to, physically and spiritually, lay aside every weight and sin. If you are physically overweight, you feel sluggish. Your friends can see the extra pounds, and every time you pass a mirror, you see them too. You know the story — your clothes fit too tight, you feel insecure, and you constantly wonder what others think of you. Finally, you decide to lose the excess body fat. At this point, you must find an effective fat loss program. As you implement this program consistently, you will see a decrease in body fat. Eventually you gain the physical results you were hoping for.

Spiritually, this same concept applies. But it is a little more difficult because spiritual weight can be hidden in your heart, where only God sees it. Well-meaning Christians often find themselves in denial over these obstacles. The spiritual weights they carry are painful to accept because they desire their actions to be pleasing to God. Although we may not acknowledge the spiritual weight, it still negatively affects us. The answer is not found in hiding the extra weight, nor in denial; the answer is found on our knees. This is where the power of exercising prayer is demonstrated.

EFFECTIVE PRAYER

Throughout history prayer has been used as an effective resource in accomplishing what otherwise could not have been achieved. We have to realize there is more than one type of prayer, but what we are discussing is the type that refuses "no" for an answer.

Many years ago the term *praying through* was used frequently in Christian circles. It has become nearly extinct in today's fast-paced society. Praying through is staying before God until you receive your answer, while at the same time trusting Him without any reservation or doubt. In many circles this type of prayer has been diminished to an ancient art that is rarely practiced.

Prayer like this requires true conviction and sincerity, without time constraints. How many people really pray with their whole hearts, believing that God is truly going to respond by answering their prayers?

Many Christians today do not pray with the same fervor that the church once did. And then we wonder why our prayers sometimes go unanswered. Because of our busy, hectic lives it is easy to make excuses not to pray the way the Bible says we should. If Daniel were alive today, he would disagree with this mentality concerning prayer. The Bible tells of a time when Daniel set his whole heart to seeking God. He *prayed through* expecting God to answer regardless of how long it took. His time of seeking God lasted twenty-one days. God answered Daniel's prayer, not because he did it for a specific length of time, but because of his commitment, his mindset, his consistency, his intensity, his motive, and his faith in God.

Jesus consistently and passionately spent time in prayer with His Father. His communication with God was so impactful that the lives around Him were changed. During His earthly ministry He taught, preached, healed the sick, and impressively enough, even raised the dead. But of all the things Jesus did that His disciples saw, there was only one thing they specifically asked Him to teach them. They said, *"Lord, teach us to pray."* The one thing they saw that was more impactful than anything else in His ministry was His prayer life. The disciples understood that what Jesus did in prayer affected His preaching, His teaching, and His ability to perform miracles. In other words, the time He spent *praying through* supplied people's needs.

Jesus is our perfect example of true prayer. He teaches us that our prayer life and relationship with God will change our own lives, and the lives of those around us.

Scripture repetitively shows that when God's people sincerely seek His face and pray, He responds by answering our prayers.

UNANSWERED PRAYER

It has been established biblically, that God answers prayer and that prayer works. So why do some Christians not receive answers to their prayers? Some would say, "I have prayed on numerous occasions and felt there was no intervention from God, so I'm not sure just how effective prayer really is."

The answer to this problem is hearing and obeying God's voice. The Bible says that the Lord's sheep hear His voice and that they won't follow anyone else. Notice, the Bible doesn't say, "Christians hear my voice." The difference is you can be a Christian and, at the same time, be a lamb, not a sheep. The lambs have to learn His voice, but the sheep know His voice. The sheep have developed intimacy in their relationship with God, so they know God hears them. Through experience and maturity, they have learned to hear His voice as well.

God receives glory when your prayers are answered. He desires to answer your prayers more than you desire to have them answered. As Christians, we should be surprised when we *don't* get an answer to our prayers, not when we do.

If your prayers go unanswered, there must be a reason. So, we are going to explore some of the possibilities for why your prayers have not been answered:

- **Lack of Faith** – Faith is not an option, but is necessary for answered prayer. We are instructed in the book of James that it is important to pray in faith or we shouldn't expect to receive anything from God. James 1:6–8 says, *"Let him ask in faith, nothing wavering. For he that wavereth is like a wave of the sea driven with the wind and tossed. For let not that man think that he shall receive anything of the Lord. A double minded man is unstable in all his ways."*

- **Unforgiveness** – Refusing to forgive someone puts a breach between you and God, making it hard to receive your answer to prayer. Matthew 6:15 says, *"If ye forgive not men their trespasses, neither will your (heavenly) Father forgive your trespasses."*

- **Pride** – Pride is a deadly threat to an effective prayer life. Pride and prayer are in direct opposition to each other. Prayer suggests a desire to be close to God, while pride creates distance from Him. Psalm 138:6 says, *"Though the Lord be high, yet hath He respect unto the lowly: but the proud He knoweth afar off."*

- **Wrong Motives** – Prayer is not just asking to see what you can get from God. The main purpose for prayer is to develop an intimate relationship with Him. Some people would be satisfied receiving from God without a relationship, which would be tragic. But you can't desire the gift without desiring the gift-giver because the gifts will soon pass away. Having a close relationship with the Lord brings true joy and eternal life that will never pass away.

- **Unrighteousness** – James 5:16 states, *"Confess your faults one to another, and pray one for another, that ye may be healed. The effectual fervent prayer of a righteous man availeth much."* We do not approach

God in our own righteousness, but we become the righteousness of God in Christ Jesus.

- **Unawareness** – In John 16:23 we read, *"Verily, verily, I say unto you, whatsoever ye shall ask the Father in my name, He will give it you."* It is important to follow the instruction of the Lord. He told us to pray in the name of Jesus. We are not going to God in our own righteousness, but in the righteousness of Jesus. This is one of the elements of effective prayer.

- **Inconsistency** – Set a daily appointment for prayer, and meet that appointment without fail. Ephesians 6:12 suggests, *"Praying always with all prayer and supplication in the Spirit."* Luke 18:1 says, *"Jesus spoke a parable unto them to this end that men ought always to pray, and not to faint."* If we are not careful, laziness, busyness, and procrastination can detour an effective prayer life.

- **Focusing on Emotions** – We can't allow our feelings to determine our prayer life because they can change from moment to moment. Our relationship with God must not be contingent on something so fickle. It needs to be based on love, commitment, and consistency.

- **Impatience** – We live in what I call a microwave society. We want things done immediately, in our own time. But God is not on our timeline. Things must be done in His time. The Bible tells us in Hebrews 10:36-37, *"Ye have need of patience, that, after ye have done the will of God, ye might receive the promise. For yet a little while, and He that shall come will come, and will not tarry."*

- **Giving Up** – Exercising the physical body only occasionally will have little to no benefit, but developing a regular habit of exercise will yield noticeable results. Over a period of time, if exercise is continued, the body will respond by becoming stronger and by losing excess body fat. Similarly, praying one time will cause very little spiritual growth. But developing a lifestyle of prayer will result in a constant growth in your spirit and will deepen your relationship with God.

If you feel you are not receiving answers to your prayers we suggest that you honestly examine your life and compare it to the previous ten suggestions. If any area of your prayer life conflicts with these suggestions, change that element and watch your spirit man grow and your relationship with God soar.

PRAYING EFFECTIVELY

Prayer is the avenue that God has chosen to draw us close to Him. Prayer is the avenue that God chose to bless his people through. Prayer is the avenue that God chose to channel faith. 2 Chronicles 7:14 says, *"If my people, which are called by my name, shall humble themselves, and pray and seek my face, and turn from their wicked ways; then will I hear from Heaven, and will forgive their sin, and will heal their land."* Prayer gives us spiritual power and strength.

The prayer portion of the Faith & Fat Loss Program is designed to help Christians reach a level of maturity in their communication with God, so their confidence will be increased that God hears them and that He desires to answer their prayers.

To assist you in developing a consistent prayer life, follow these suggestions:

- Prayer is not a thought, but a conversation with God. Prayer was not intended to be a formality or a ritual, but a sincere conversation with your heavenly Father.

- It is important in developing an effective prayer life to know and pray God's Word – this is a safety parameter (for an example on how to use God's Word in prayer see the chapter on God's word). God Himself wants us to pray His word. The Holy Spirit will confirm His word and bring it to pass. Last, but not least, His word is a written will for our lives which is our inheritance.

- Our thoughts and feelings are solidified by the words we speak. We are made in the image of God; therefore, we have some of His attributes. God never created anything without first speaking. This same principle of expressing through words has been given to us for prayer.

- Prayer is a powerful tool that God has placed at our disposal. If we truly comprehend the effect our prayers have on our lives and on earthly circumstances, we would likely pray more earnestly, more consistently, and more effectively. James 5:17 says, *"Elias was a man subject to like passions as we are, and he prayed earnestly that it might not rain: and it rained not on the earth by the space of three years and six months."* We would do well to follow the example of Elijah, who believed that his prayers had the power to cause change in earthly circumstances.

- There is no better way to learn how to pray than to pray.

In learning the art of effective prayer, it is important to realize that we stand not on our feet; but on our knees. True strength is found when we bend our knees and bow our hearts. **You can be confident there is power on your knees!**

PRAYER AND MEMORIZATION STUDY SCHEDULE

A Prayer and Memorization/Word Study Consecration Chart can be found in the Exhibit section of the book. Below is an example of a completed chart to help you develop your own schedule. The chart includes both spiritual nutrition (study of God's Word, which is your scripture memorization) and spiritual exercise (prayer). This tool will help you stay consistent in your prayer life, both during the "spiritual detox" and beyond. At the bottom of the chart, there is a space to list things that deserve your consistent attention on which you pray for daily. While on the Faith & Fat Loss Program, spend fifteen minutes a day in prayer and fifteen minute studying scripture. This is essential to reaching your ultimate goal of permanent fat loss and true transformation.

Prayer and Memorization/Word Study Chart

	Memorization & Word Study Appointment	Memorization & Word Study Attained	Prayer Appointment	Prayer Attained
Sunday	8:00 - 8:15a.m. (15 minutes)	Minutes 30	8:15 - 8:30a.m. (15 minutes)	Minutes 15
Monday	6:00 - 6:15 a.m.	Minutes 30	6:15 - 6:30 a.m.	Minutes 15
Tuesday	6:00 - 6:15 a.m.	Minutes 15	6:15 - 6:30 a.m.	Minutes 15
Wednesday	6:00 - 6:15 a.m.	Minutes 30	6:15 - 6:30 a.m.	Minutes 15
Thursday	6:00 - 6:15 a.m.	Minutes 30	6:15 - 6:30 a.m.	Minutes 15
Friday	6:00 - 6:15 a.m.	Minutes 15	6:15 - 6:30 a.m.	Minutes 15
Saturday	10:00 - 10:15 a.m.	Minutes 15	10:15 - 10:30 a.m.	Minutes 15
WEEKLY TOTALS	1 hr. 45 min.	2 HOURS 45 MINUTES	1 hr. 45 min.	1 HOUR 45 MINUTES

Prayer List:

SELF:

LOVED ONES:

OTHER:

At the bottom of the chart, write the names of people you want to pray for during your prayer times and specific things to pray about for them. For yourself, you may choose to pray for strength, courage, faith, discipline, or consistency to achieve fat loss. List friends, relatives, and loved ones who need prayer. Include your pastor, missionaries, and government leaders.

Also, make a list of specific things in your life that deserve your attention. For example, if someone has caused a soul wound in your life, pray for complete forgiveness of the perpetrator.

PRAYER REQUESTS

In the Faith & Fat Loss website we have established an online prayer community for the purpose of asking God to strengthen those who are going through physical and spiritual detox, as well as those who are struggling with soul wounds. We pray for all those who desire to decrease body fat and experience a true transformation. To enter your prayer requests, or to be a prayer warrior, visit our Website at www.faithandfatloss.com

Chapter 17

SUPPLEMENTATION:

Physical and Spiritual

Physical and Spiritual Supplementation is a vital part of the Faith & Fat Loss Program. The word *supplement* means "in addition to," not "in place of." Supplementation has become necessary because many of the nutrients required for health, and vitality are missing.

Some of the vitamins and minerals no longer occur naturally in our food sources in the quantities they once did. To add insult to injury, many of the foods we ingest are loaded with chemicals and toxins. This is why good nutritional supplementation is essential in acquiring optimal health and fat loss.

Spiritually, we have a similar necessity for supplementation. Our spiritual nourishment is derived from the Word of God. When the Word of God is watered down or compromised by man's inaccurate interpretation or opinion, it becomes toxic to our spirit man because it's no longer God's Word. The spiritual supplements in this program are designed to direct us away from the world's toxic influence and lead us back to the authentic Word of God

The supplements advocated by this program are designed to help you detoxify the physical and spiritual body and acquire the healthy balance God intended. The Word of God stands alone and needs no supplementation, just as the foods originally created by God needed no supplementation. The necessity of supplements for both our physical and spiritual food was caused only through man's interference.

Physical Supplements

Supplementation is a vast and complicated world within itself. Through the Faith & Fat Loss Supplementation Program, we have removed the guesswork in finding effective supplementation. **I have created, for this program, high quality supplements to obtain maximum results in healthy fat loss.** These products were originally produced solely for my personal use as a professional competitor. But these remarkable products are now available for consumers who want to decrease body fat. The Faith & Fat Loss supplement line will help your body better absorb nutrients, assist in muscle growth, and help increase energy. These products also have the essential nutrients needed for wellness, fat loss, and longevity.

Thousands of supplements are being sold today. Each one claims to facilitate a particular need in the human body. In my extensive research I have found that some of these supplements produce results, but many just don't. This puts the consumer in a precarious position. They want to purchase supplements that will meet their needs, but they have no way of knowing whether a particular supplement has the proper quantity and quality of each ingredient necessary to produce real results for them.

The supplement portion of the Faith & Fat Loss Program relieves you from the responsibility of having to spend hours of study to determine the effectiveness of each supplement.

I have produced the Faith & Fat Loss products with the following in mind:

- The ingredients in each product must meet the standards of accurate, proven, scientific research necessary to achieve maximum results.
- In developing these products, I used the most effective high-quality ingredients, in the proper quantities, to accomplish long-term fat loss and optimal health.
- The quality of our products have not been compromised by using insufficient sub-standard ingredients.

- In order to be successful with a supplementation regimen consistency is required. So this program was designed to easily facilitate the average lifestyle. The supplements are designed to be taken during times of the day that are convenient for today's active lifestyle, rather than throughout the day.

The following are three supplements that I recommend to aid you in maximizing your fat loss results:

Ron Williams Trace Minerals

Minerals affect every function of every cell in the body, including the thought process, eye movement, and heartbeat.

The body cannot perform properly without a good source of pure ionic trace minerals. The body is bio-electrically conducted, which means all of your physical movements are controlled by a brain-nerve connection through the conduit of minerals. For example, when you stand up your brain sends a signal, not to the muscles in the legs, but through the nerves attached to the leg muscles. Only then does movement take place. Without a proper mineral balance, your body receives diluted signals. An improper mineral balance can contribute to depression, ADHD, and an overstressed endocrine system, which will dramatically affect your ability to decrease body fat. Our mineral deficient toxic society makes a high-quality source of ionic trace minerals absolutely necessary.

Ron Williams Trace Minerals provide a proper balance of these life-giving nutrients. They allow for effective repair and function of each cell and facilitate the body's nervous system. Ron Williams Trace Minerals are designed for maximum absorption into the cells.

One of the least expensive, most productive, quickest, easiest things that you can do to decrease body fat is to change the type of water you drink. Distilled water is pure water, which is H2O plus nothing. Tap water, on the other hand, is H2O plus a small amount of minerals and fat loss resistant chemicals, which leads to excess body fat. The distilled water does not have any minerals and so must be fortified with ionic trace minerals. In the Faith & Fat Loss program we recommend that you drink 64 oz. of distilled water daily with approximately 30 drops of minerals added. The minerals are essential for the 21-Day Jump Start, but we recommend that in order to continue and maintain fat loss this should become a permanent part of your new lifestyle.

For more information on minerals and pure water, visit our Website at www.faithandfatloss.com.

Ron Williams Fat Burn "5"

With all of the ineffective and dangerous fat burning products and ingredients on the market, we have searched in-depth to find ingredients that will increase health while producing maximum fat loss. Fat Burn "5" is a completely natural, high-intensity, healthy fat metabolizer. Taken along with a proper nutrition and exercise program, it will contribute to a significant decrease in body fat, improve your overall health, and increase longevity. It helps reduce body fat through a combination of five potent ingredients. Each of these ingredients has its own unique pathway of reducing body fat.

The following is an explanation of how each ingredient works to assist with decreasing body fat.

L-Carnitine – L-Carnitine is an amino acid that has been scientifically proven to move fat out of the fat cell to be burned as energy. In combination with chromium it helps to form the transport system used to move fat into the mitochondria (engines of the body found in the muscle) to be used as energy. Without this essential amino acid, your body will not decrease body fat at the same rate. L-Carnitine also helps to increase muscle endurance.

Chromium – Chromium is one of the most depleted micronutrients in the western diet. One of its primary functions is to facilitate calories into the muscle cell to be burned as energy. If your body does not have proper amounts of chromium the calories cannot enter the muscle cell; instead, they are reverted to the liver and stored as fat in the fat cell. This leaves the body depleted of energy, which causes cravings for starches, simple sugars, chocolate, and other foods that are counterproductive to your fat loss goals. A lack of chromium causes low energy, increased cravings, decreased muscle size, and excess body fat. Chromium reduces cravings by stabilizing the blood sugar level. This mineral can be toxic if too much is taken, or if an incorrect source is consumed, so you must be careful when supplementing. The type of chromium in Fat Burn "5" is niacin-bound, which is an extremely safe form of chromium.

Eleutherococcus Senticosus – Eleutherococcus senticosus is a powerful tonic herb with an impressive range of health benefits. It is used as a treatment in times of stress, pressure, and depression. During stressful situations the adrenal glands release cortisol and adrenaline. If the energy created by cortisol is not used, it will be converted to fat and stored in the fat cells, mainly in the abdominal and hip area. Eleutherococcus slows down this process and allows a more economical and efficient release of these hormones. This provides two benefits: sparing the exhaustion of the adrenal glands and curbing the body's natural response of producing excess body fat. Eleutherococcus also causes the body to burn fat rather than carbohydrates during exercise, increases oxygen in the body, and causes a surplus of energy.

Iodine – The thyroid gland controls the metabolism, which means it determines how much energy is being used by the body through daily activity. If your metabolism is high, your body produces more heat, causing more calories to be burned; if your metabolism is low, your body requires fewer calories to function. Without iodine, the thyroid cannot function properly. One of the main culprits of low thyroid hormones is lack of iodine. Low iodine equates to excess body fat. In today's society, not only are we deficient in iodine, our environment is filled with halogens and estrogen mimickers (See Chapter 5). These chemicals compete not only with the thyroid, but also with iodine in occupying space in the fat cells. If the fat cell is occupied with estrogen mimickers and halogens, continual fat gain is inevitable. If iodine is in the fat cells, fat loss is likely.

Vitamin C (Sodium Ascorbate) – If your desire is to lose fat, the type of vitamin C you consume is critical. The acid form, ascorbic acid, is an inferior type of Vitamin C and can actually contribute to fat gain. The alkaline form, sodium ascorbate, is more costly than the acid form, but it is the type of vitamin C that contributes to fat loss. Without adequate amounts of vitamin C you are more apt to put on extra body fat. And studies show those who have the lowest levels of vitamin C have the highest amounts of body fat. Individuals with adequate vitamin C oxidize 30 percent more fat during exercise than individuals with low levels of vitamin C. This means that if you are vitamin C depleted, you have decreased your body's ability to rid itself of excess body fat. Adequate amounts of the proper type of vitamin C in your diet, combined with sensible eating and exercise, can be a good safeguard against putting weight back on. Vitamin C (Sodium Ascorbate) works synergistically with the other ingredients in Fat Burn "5". It works with L-Carnitine to oxidize fat in the body. It also increases the absorption of chromium. Vitamin C is also an antioxidant that works with eleutherococcus to heal the adrenal glands, enhance the immune system, and decrease body fat.

Ron Williams Food Complex

This product is a natural, high energy, protein food complex. A food complex is a meal replacement that contains a balance of protein, carbohydrates, and essential fatty acids (EFA). The Ron Williams Food Complex is an elite product because of the unique formulation of nutrients that have been combined to create a high-quality nutritional supplement that is hard to find. The distinct difference of this product is the source and quality of the all-natural, organic ingredients. This food complex combines two of nature's most complete and dependable sources of protein: milk and eggs. The uniqueness of these ingredients are that the chickens are vegetarian fed and range free, and neither the cows nor the chickens have been injected with bovine growth hormones or antibiotics. Also, the milk has not been homogenized. As the essential fatty acid, this product also includes the highest-quality of lecithin and phosphatidyl choline. Combined with an exercise program and good nutrition these ingredients work to lower cholesterol and triglycerides (blood fat), increase metabolism (which aids in fat loss), and to aid in reversing some of the effects of estrogen dominance, halogens, and other toxins.

The Food Complex is a complete meal that can be used as a substitute for one of your daily meals (breakfast, lunch, snack, or dinner).

More than 21 Simple Ways to Lose Body Fat

I have also written a book called *More than 21 Simple Ways to Lose Body Fat*. It provides simple, practical strategies that have been scientifically proven to decrease body fat—safely and effectively. This book was written from 25 years of practical experience and scientific research. The strategies in the *More than 21 Simple Ways* book are easy to understand and to apply. And we have given more than 21 effective tools that can be used as a supplement to enhance your fat loss as you are engaged in the Faith & Fat Loss lifestyle.

SPIRITUAL SUPPLEMENTS

Whatever we do on the inside will reveal itself on the outside. The Word of God says it like this, "*that which is done in the dark shall be brought to light.*" The work we do internally, to improve our souls, will be revealed externally in our actions and in our physical bodies.

The spiritual supplementation in the Faith & Fat Loss program has been provided to enhance your awareness of God's desire for you to be all that you can be, physically and spiritually. These tools will aid you in understanding what the Word of God has to say about health, longevity, fat loss, and spiritual transformation.

Transformation Success Journal

Life's triumphs and struggles are hard to remember after they have passed. Journaling helps us recall the struggles God carried us through. As we think back on those times, we begin to realize we can accomplish difficult tasks. As God's Word says, *we can do all things through Christ who strengthens us.*

Journaling can also be a reminder of your commitment to Scripture and prayer, which can help keep you on track in those areas. As you journey toward true transformation, there will come a time when the things that have changed become permanent because of God's influence – this is true transformation.

Journaling is a personal experience that cannot be bound to specific criteria. However, I offer the following suggestions to help you successfully track your spiritual and physical progress:

- Record your daily prayers.
- Record the answers to prayer.
- Write down and study your memorization Scriptures.
- Document your feelings and emotions.
- Track your weight
- Describe your spiritual breakthroughs.
- Express your struggles.
- Track the dates, times, and types of exercise.
- Journal your diet and nutrition plan.

There are many traits that successful people have. One of those traits is that they write down and track their goals, desires, and successes. We have provided for you in the back of the book a 21-Day Journal to track your feelings, struggles, successes, and goals during the 21-Day Jump Start. This will create a habit that you can take into the continuation phase of your journey.

Faith & Fat Loss Scripture Memorization Cards

The Faith & Fat Loss Scripture Memorization Cards are a compilation of Scripture verses. The cards have the memorization verse on one side and an explanation of how the scripture pertains to fat loss and transformation on the other side. These cards are an exceptional tool that will aid you in increasing your knowledge and understanding of God's Word, as well as increasing your prayer life, furthering your walk with God, and achieving your ultimate fat loss goals.

The Scripture Memorization Cards will:

- Empower you against attacks of the enemy.
- Further your understanding of God's Word.
- Teach you to use the Word of God as an effective weapon.
- Increase your spiritual maturity.
- Encourage and strengthen you.
- Teach you to use Scripture to bring comfort.
- Increase your faith.
- Help you develop discipline.
- Draw you closer to God.
- Maximize your ability to achieve transformation.

The *Faith & Fat Loss Scripture Memorization Cards* can be found at www.faithandfatloss.com.

Faith & Fat Loss Website

The Faith & Fat Loss Website was designed as a tool and a supplement to help you on your journey to lose body fat, increase your spiritual awareness, and strengthen your relationship with God. Our goal is to minister to the whole person – spiritually, physically, and emotionally. The Word of God tells us in Hosea 4:6 that God's people are destroyed for lack of knowledge. This site will give you the knowledge and assistance you need to lose the unwanted body fat, and will help guide you gently through the process of overcoming spiritual and physical hindrances. Ultimately, you will have increased self-esteem, become physically and spiritually fit, shed the excess physical and spiritual weight, and develop a more intimate relationship with God.

You will find the following tools that will help and support you in reaching your fat loss and transformation goals:

- Personal balanced meal plans
- Recipes
- Exercise tutorials
- Progress charts
- Special forums and blogs
- Ron Williams personalized support and prayers through webinars and email blasts
- Product discounts
- And more!

Physical and spiritual supplementation should not only be considered a luxury, but a necessity if your goal is to successfully decrease body fat, enhance your health and longevity, and acquire true transformation. Don't minimize your need for quality supplementation if you want to maximize your long-term results. With the Faith & Fat Loss program, we have developed supplements to assure your success.

I want to welcome you to the Faith & Fat Loss family!

Chapter 18

MEASURE YOUR PROGRESS

One of the fundamentals of success is measuring your progress. In the Faith & Fat Loss program we have chosen several different tools to give you a precise record of your physical and spiritual advancement.

There are many benefits to measuring your progress. The first is that your progress becomes tangible, something you can pinpoint. It removes the frustration of guessing and wondering if you are truly getting results. Next, measuring will hold you accountable. Another benefit is that it allows you to see yourself for who you are, and your progress for what it really is.

The success rate for individuals who accurately measure their progress is much higher than for those who don't. You will need comprehensive tools to measure your progress, which are unbiased and based on facts. An accurate form of measurement is not something that is subjective. It is not the eyes of loved ones who desire to see you reach your goals. Although, they may be a terrific source of encouragement their assessment of your progress could be biased. Your own eyes aren't much better. Since you see yourself on a daily basis, it's hard to see gradual changes.

It's important to have an accurate measuring stick to track your progress. In the Faith & Fat Loss program I have chosen the following tools to give you a precise record of your physical and spiritual advancement:

Physical Progress:
- Before and after pictures
- Weight
- Body measurements

Spiritual Progress:
- Scripture memorization
- Prayer

If you accurately follow this program, and continue with it, you will be successful. These measuring tools will motivate and encourage you to stay on course.

Measuring your physical progress:

BEFORE AND AFTER PICTURES

You've probably heard the saying "A picture speaks louder than a thousand words." This couldn't be any more evident than with before and after pictures.

One of my favorite illustrations of this is a girl that participated in the Faith & Fat Loss program who had a deep soul wound and an excessive amount of fat to lose. She progressed tremendously, but felt discouraged because as she saw herself on a daily basis it was hard for her to recognize how many ounces and inches she had actually lost. She didn't realize that the ounces lost turned into pounds, and the pounds lost turned into a decrease in clothing size. But when the "after" picture was taken and compared to her "before" picture, her discouragement that could have lead to giving up and leaving the program turned into excitement and a determination to continue striving toward the goals she had originally set. She saw visually the progress she had made when she looked at the pictures

If done properly, losing fat is a gradual lasting process. Losing a pound or two of excess body fat in a week's time is quite substantial, but not very noticeable to a person who is hard on themselves. Most of us are our own worst critics—I know that I am. By taking accurate pictures you will have a true visual measurement of your progress.

Following are some guidelines to follow when taking before, during, and after pictures.

1. Take all pictures in the same place.
2. Take pictures in lighting that reveals details, and make sure the lighting is the same each time. The lighting will cause the pictures to vary somewhat as far as seeing definition or cellulite.
3. Take all pictures from the same distance. It's best to mark the spot.
4. If possible take all the pictures with the same camera.
5. Relax during all picture-taking sessions. Holding your stomach in may give you a better appearance, but it will distort the reality of your true progress in the next set of pictures.
6. Take pictures, the first and last day of the 21-Day Jump Start and then again every 30 days.

Take at least six pictures each time: one of the front, one of the back, and one of each side, capturing the whole body (from head to toe), and two close-ups of your most unappealing areas that you most desire to improve.

BODY WEIGHT

Body weight is the least vital of the measuring tools for several reasons. One reason is that your body is made up of 60 to 70 percent water. Water weight tends to fluctuate, from two to seven pounds, with even minor changes in your activities or what you eat. Another issue with measuring body weight is that some people become so obsessed with the scales that it turns into a discouragement or a distraction.

Measuring your body weight can be an effective tool if not over used. Weigh yourself on a scale before you start the fat-loss program, to give yourself a starting measurement. Then weigh again after the 21-Day Jump Start. Weigh periodically throughout the continuation and maintenance program.

BODY MEASUREMENTS

There are thirteen critical measuring points that will give you an accurate analysis of your progress. In measuring the body, you must be careful to measure accurately because it is easy to get a false calculation if no systematic method is applied. We will use the thirteen measuring points to determine inches gained or lost. With this technique, each area will be measured until the largest area is found. This will take a number of measurements. After the largest area is found, measure the largest area three times. The largest measurement will be recorded.

If you measure a body part incorrectly, you may see a wide discrepancy when you measure the same body part the next time. If you don't measure the largest circumference on the first measurement and the next time you measure you do measure the largest area it will appear as though you did not lose any inches, when you actually did.

Taking three measurements for each body part decreases the margin for error. If you find the largest area of a particular body part and measure it three times, you will have a more accurate reading.

Here are some guidelines for measuring each body part accurately:

1. Make sure the measuring tape is taut when it touches the surface of the skin, but that it does not make an impression. This must be consistent each time you measure.
2. Carefully follow the directions below for each measuring site.
3. Have a trusted individual take measurements for you. If possible, have the same person measure you each time.
4. Relax the abdominal area and breathe normally when being measured. If you hold your abs in the first time you measure, and relax the second time you measure; although you may have lost inches, the second reading may appear to be the same or larger than the first, when it is actually smaller.
5. Take measurements the first and last day of the 21 Day Jump Start and then again every 30 days.

This chart can assist you in keeping a record of your progress.

MEASURE YOUR SUCCESS

Body Measurement Chart

	1st	2nd	3rd	4th	5th
Date:					
Weight:					
Calves	R	R	R	R	R
	L	L	L	L	L
Thighs	R	R	R	R	R
	L	L	L	L	L
Hips					
Glutes					
Lower Abdominals					
1" Above Navel					
Back and Chest					
Arms	R	R	R	R	R
	L	L	L	L	L
Shoulders					
Neck					
TOTAL:					

For your own Body Measurement Chart
see exhibit 5 in the back of the book.

DIRECTIONS FOR MEASURING EACH POINT

Below are instructions for your trusted individual to follow when measuring each of your body parts. (To avoid the confusion of gender-neutral plural pronouns and the awkwardness of *him/her* pronouns, I will refer to your trusted individual as a male.)

Measuring Point No. 1 and 2 – Calf

Measuring point No. 1 and 2 is the calf muscle. Remember to measure both calf muscles. Face your trusted individual placing your left leg slightly in front of your body distributing nearly all of your weight on your right leg. Lift your left heel, leaving the ball of your foot on the floor. In this position, have your trusted individual take three measurements of the largest area of your calf muscle. Record the largest reading on your chart. Repeat the process for the right leg.

Measuring Point No. 3 and 4 - Thigh

Measuring point No. 3 and 4 is the largest part of the thigh (upper leg). Stand in the same position as you did for measuring the calf muscle. Have your trusted individual put the tape measure behind your thigh at the base of the gluts (buttocks) and bring both ends of the tape to the front. Find the largest area by taking several readings. Then measure three times and record the largest reading. Repeat for the other leg.

Measuring Point No. 5 - Hips

Measuring point No. 5 is the hip area located outside both legs level with where the gluts and hamstrings (back of thigh) connect. Stand with your feet and heels together. Have your trusted individual stand to your side placing the measuring tape around your hips, pulling both sides of the tape toward him until they come together. Take a number of readings to find the largest area and then measure three times, and record the largest reading.

Measuring Point No. 6 - Gluts

Measuring point No. 6 is the gluts (buttocks). Have your trusted individual stand to your side. He will place the measuring tape above your hip area, keeping the tape horizontal to the floor, and pulling the tape toward him until both ends come together. Find the largest reading, measure three times, and record the largest measurement.

Measuring Point No. 7 – Lower Abdomen

Measuring point No. 7 is the lower abdominal area. Have your trusted individual stand at your side. Have him reach to the opposite side of your body, place the tape above your hips, and pull it around the largest part of your lower abdominal area, keeping the tape horizontal to the floor. Find the largest part of the abdominal area, take three measurements and record the largest.

Measuring Point No. 8 – 1" Above the Navel

Measuring Point No. 8 is one inch above the navel. Have your trusted individual put his finger one inch above your navel, then reach to the opposite side of your body and bring the tape across the measuring point. Find the largest area and make sure the tape does not go into any creases. Find the largest circumference (1 inch above the navel), then take three measurements and record the largest.

Measuring Point No. 9 – Back and Chest

Measuring Point No. 9 is the back and chest. Have your trusted individual stand behind you and place the measuring tape in front of you. Put the tape in the center of your chest or on the nipple line. Have your trusted individual pull the tape toward him tautly. Drop your arms, pulling your shoulders forward as far as possible, spreading your back. Make sure the tape is not trapped under your armpits forcing a false measurement. Have your trusted individual bring both ends of the tape together to take up the slack. Repeat this process until you find the largest circumference of the upper back and chest. Take three measurements and record the largest.

Measuring Point No. 10 and 11 – Arms (Biceps)

Measuring Point No. 10 and 11 are the arms. Stand in front of your trusted individual. Raise one arm, with your triceps horizontal to the floor. Contract your biceps muscle by pulling your fist close to your shoulder. Have your trusted individual place the tape at the peak of your biceps and around the largest part of your triceps. Find the largest measurement, take three readings, and record the largest. Repeat this process for the other arm.

Measuring Point No. 12 - Shoulders

Measuring Point No. 12 will be the shoulders width and thickness. Stand to the side of your trusted individual and have him reach with the measuring tape to your opposite shoulder. Have him pull both sides of the tape toward him until they meet, making sure the tape is horizontal to the floor. Find the largest part of the shoulders, then take three readings, and record the largest measurement.

Measuring Point No. 13 – Neck

Measuring Point No. 13 is the neck. Stand beside your trusted individual. Have him reach with the measuring tape to the opposite side of your neck. Keep the tape horizontal to the floor. Have him pull both sides of the tape toward him until they meet. Find the largest part of the neck, take three measurements, and record the largest measurement.

If the measurements are done properly the first time, after the first twenty-one days you should see a significant difference in inches lost.

Measuring your Spiritual Progress:

We have set-up the following guidelines for measuring your spiritual progress because if you are not progressing spiritually, soul wounds and stumbling blocks will keep you captive and prevent you from obtaining permanent success. As you grow spiritually, you will have the strength to do what is necessary to progress physically. In other words, what takes place on the inside (your spiritual body) will manifest itself on the outside (your physical body).

Scripture Memorization

The Word of God is a spiritual weapon you can use to increase your faith and to fight against anything that is contrary to God's plan and purpose for your life. The enemy's job is to keep you from truly understanding it. So, as a Christian, it is important to apply this weapon (the Word of God) to overcome all stumbling blocks that may try to hinder you.

The Bible contains knowledge pertaining to all natural circumstances, as well as spiritual affairs. Whatever situation you're in, you can find the answer in God's Word. True success comes from believing, knowing, and applying the Word of God.

Joshua 1:8 states, *"This book of the law shall not depart out of thy mouth; but thou shalt meditate therein day and night, that thou mayest observe to do according to all that is written therein: for then thou shalt make thy way prosperous, and then thou shalt have good success."* God commanded Joshua to perform a task that was against his nature. Joshua resisted because of fear. The Lord then gave him the solution to obtain success, not just over fear, but over every area of life.

Here are a few indicators you can use to measure your progress in the area of Scripture memorization:

1. In times of stress or pressure, your response will become less carnal and noticeably more spiritual if you are continuously renewing your mind with the Word of God.

2. When you're facing a problem, the Scriptures you have memorized flood your mind and the appropriate solution becomes clear.

3. In times of spiritual, emotional, and dietary weakness, it becomes second nature to pray for strength using your memorized Scriptures.

These are good indicators that you are progressing and being successful with your memorization scriptures. The Word of God will strengthen you in times of need when you have hidden it in your heart through memorization. First John 2:14 states, *"I have written unto you young men, because ye are strong, and the Word of God abideth in you."*

PRAYER

The Faith & Fat Loss spiritual exercise program is designed to teach you how to pray, enhance your spiritual walk with God, and make prayer a way of life. You can measure your progress in prayer by the following:

- **How effortless prayer becomes.** Prayer is not always an easy task, especially if you haven't done it much. First of all, it is communication with a Spiritual Being who can't be seen when we are accustomed to talking with people who respond immediately. Sometimes you may feel like you are doing all the talking in a one-sided conversation. Secondly, when you begin your prayer life the words may not come very easily and you might have to search for words rather than just relaxing and communicating. As you progress, prayer will become more comfortable and fluid.
- **Increased confidence that God not only can, but that He will answer your prayers.** As your prayer life progresses when problems arise prayer becomes second nature and your first line of defense.
- **It becomes more natural to trust in God.** God says cast all of your cares on Him and the way you do this is through prayer. As you grow in your prayer life you will find that it is much easier to turn over those things that were once hard to impossible to trust and release to God.
- **By allowing the Holy Spirit to be your comforter.** As you fully commit yourself to prayer it becomes more effortless to exchange the comfort of food for the comfort of the Holy Spirit.

By following the Faith & Fat Loss spiritual exercise program you can be assured that your relationship with God will deepen.

Chapter 19

THE POWER OF YOUR WILL

"WILL thou be made whole?"—John 5:6

You have come to the place of accepting a call to action, which requires your *will*. Don't take this word *will* lightly. It is a tremendous gift God has given you that must be activated to complete your true transformation.

There are many definitions of the word *will*; such as, "to yearn for or desire." But we confuse these definitions with the amazing gift that God has given us. The word *will* that we are speaking of is a spiritual gift that is a determined command of oneself to fulfill a commitment. It is a verbal announcement that is declared or decreed in the heart.

Finally, when you use the word *will* it can be a foretelling of future events in your life. The only thing lacking to be successful is the time required for the event to come to pass.

Your *will* and your ability to decree a thing are interchangeable, as found in Job 22:28: *"Thou shalt also decree [will] a thing, and it shall be established unto thee (you)."* When you decree a thing according to God's desire for your life by activating your *will*, this Scripture says you will succeed in whatever you choose to do.

Consider making the following decrees for yourself:

- I *will* decrease body fat.
- I *will* overcome my soul wounds.
- I *will* allow God to knock down the walls of limitation.
- I *will* achieve God's purpose for my life.
- I *will* receive true transformation.

If you agree with these five "I wills," I recommend that you sign the decree below.

"I (name) decree (or will) to implement the Faith & Fat Loss Program for the purpose of decreasing body fat, overcoming soul wounds, knocking down the walls of limitation, achieving God's purpose for my life, and receiving true transformation."

_____

Signature/Date

Section V

Additional Tools for your Success

21- Day
Transformation

---

*Success
Journal*

"Trust in the Lord with all your heart; and lean not unto your own understanding. In all thy ways acknowledge Him, and He shall direct thy paths." —**Proverbs 3:5-6**

–Day 1–

"If my people, which are called by my name, shall humble themselves, and pray, and seek my face, and turn from their wicked ways; then will I hear from heaven, and will forgive their sin, and will heal their land." —**2 Chronicles 7:14**

—Day 2—

"The Lord is my light and my salvation; whom shall I fear? The Lord is the strength of my life; of whom shall I be afraid?"
—Psalm 27:1

—Day 3—

"And be not conformed to this world: but be transformed by the renewing of your mind, that you may prove what is that good, and acceptable, and perfect, will of God." —**Romans 12:2**

–*Day 4*–

"One day Jesus told his disciples a story to show that they should always pray and never give up." —**Luke 18:1 (NLT)**

–*Day* 5–

But my God shall supply all your need according to His riches in glory by Christ Jesus. —**Philippians 4:19**

—Day 6—

"I can do all things through Christ which strengthens me."
—Philippians 4:13

–*Day 7*–

_____

_____

_____

_____

_____

_____

_____

_____

_____

_____

_____

_____

_____

_____

_____

_____

_____

_____

_____

_____

_____

_____

_____

_____

_____

_____

_____

"This book of the law shall not depart out of thy mouth; but thou shalt meditate therein day and night, that thou mayest observe to do according to all that is written therein: for then thou shalt make thy way prosperous, and then thou shalt have good success." —Joshua 1:8

—Day 8—

"So then faith cometh by hearing, and hearing by the Word of God."
—Romans 10:17

—Day 9—

"So that we may boldly say, The Lord is me helper, and I will not fear what man shall do unto me." —**Hebrews 13:6**

–*Day* 10–

"Have not I commanded thee? Be strong and of a good courage; be not afraid, neither be thou dismayed: for the Lord thy God is with thee whithersoever thou go." —**Joshua 1:9**

—Day 11—

_____

_____

_____

_____

_____

_____

_____

_____

_____

_____

_____

_____

_____

_____

_____

_____

_____

_____

_____

_____

_____

_____

_____

_____

"For I know the thoughts that I think toward you, saith the Lord, thoughts of peace, and not of evil, to give you an expected end."
—*Jeremiah 29:11*

—Day 12—

"Know you not that they which run in a race run all, but one receiveth the prize? So run, that you may obtain."
—1 Corinthians 9:24

–Day 13–

_____

_____

_____

_____

_____

_____

_____

_____

_____

_____

_____

_____

_____

_____

_____

_____

_____

_____

_____

_____

_____

_____

_____

_____

_____

"For the joy of the Lord is your strength."
—Nehemiah 8:10

–*Day 14*–

"And Jesus answered him, saying, it is written, That man shall not live by bread alone, but by every word of God."
—Luke 4:4

—Day 15—

"What? Know you not that your body is the temple of the Holy Ghost which is in you, which you have of God, and you are not your own?"
—1 Corinthians 6:19

–Day 16–

_____
_____
_____
_____
_____
_____
_____
_____
_____
_____
_____
_____
_____
_____
_____
_____
_____
_____
_____
_____
_____
_____
_____
_____
_____

"I will praise You, for I am fearfully and wonderfully made;
Marvelous are your works, and that my soul knows very well."
—Psalm 139:14

—Day 17—

"Wait on the Lord; be of good courage, and He shall strengthen your heart; Wait, I say, on the Lord!"
—Psalm 27:14

—Day 18—

"But I discipline my body and bring it into subjection, lest, when I have preached to others, I myself should become disqualified."
—*1 Corinthians 9:27*

—Day 19—

"Many are the afflictions of the righteous: but the Lord delivers him out of them all." —**Psalm 34:19**

–*Day 20*–

"You shall not fear them: for the Lord your God he shall fight for you."
—Deuteronomy 3:22

–Day 21–

EXHIBIT 1

MSG and MSG Derivatives

Disguised Names for MSG

Monsodium Glutamate

Glutamate

Calcium Caseinate

Monopotassium Glutamate

Yeast Nutrient

Yeast Extract

Hydrolyzed Corn Gluten

Natrium Glutamate

Glutamic Acid

Gelatin

Sodium Caseinate

Textured Protein

Autolyzed Yeast

Yeast Food

Hydrolyzed Protein

Other Sources of MSG or Free Glutamates

Maltodextrin

Malt Extract

Soy Protein Isolate

Bouillon and Broth

Soy Sauce

Soy Sauce Extract

Natural Chicken Flavoring Stock

Whey Protein Concentrate

Barley Malt

Protease

All Modified Enzymes

Seasonings (the word)

Flavors and Flavorings

Citric Acid

Malt Flavoring

Natural Pork Flavoring

Natural Beef Flavoring

Soy Protein

Whey Protein

Carrageenan

Ultra-Pasteurized

Soy Protein Concentrate

Pectin

All Fermented

Whey Protein Isolate

Natural Flavors

Be very careful of fractionated proteins and vegetables, these are normally MSG derivatives (ex., Pea Protein or Corn Protein).

EXHIBIT 2

Becoming a Soul Survivor

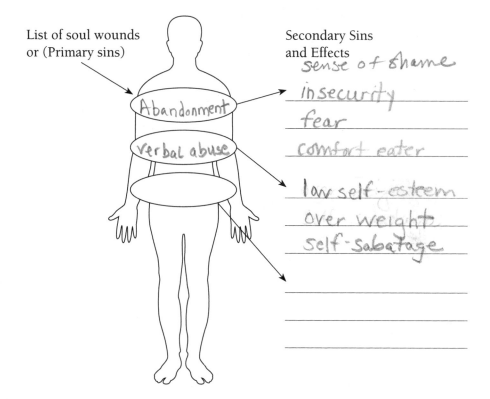

List of soul wounds
or (Primary sins)

Secondary Sins
and Effects

sense of shame
insecurity
fear
comfort eater

low self-esteem
over weight
self-sabatage

Abandonment

Verbal abuse

By prayerfully going through this exercise, you will experience God's healing touch from these painful wounds and the sins and effects associated with them. Examine yourself and identify the soul wounds and record them in the diagram. With every soul wound there are secondary sins and effects, identify these and record them as well. Now you are able to complete the 5 RE's of Soul Surviving on Page 90.

EXHIBIT 3A

21 Day Jump Start - Daily Food Chart

	Breakfast	Snack	Lunch	Snack	Dinner	Snack
Protein						
Essential Fatty Acid						
Fibrous Carbs.						
Starchy Carbs.					Not allowed after 3 p.m.	Not allowed after 3 p.m.
Simple Carbs.	Not allowed during the 21 Day Jump Start!					

Notice during the last two meals that your only options for carbohydrates are fibrous carbohydrates. Fibrous carbs are high in fiber and low in calories. At night, the body is preparing to go into a semi-hibernation state and the metabolism slows. During this time excess carbohydrates can easily be converted into fat. Make sure you eat your last meal a minimum of two hours before bed.

EXHIBIT 3B

Continuation & Maintenance - Daily Food Chart

	Breakfast	Snack	Lunch	Snack	Dinner	Snack
Protein						
Essential Fatty Acid						
Fibrous Carbs.						
Starchy Carbs.					Not allowed after 3 p.m.	
Simple Carbs.					Not allowed after 3 p.m.	

It is wise to always carry healthy snacks with you. Protein shakes, cheese sticks, raw nuts, and fruit are just a few good examples to keep handy just in case the unexpected happens; such as, getting caught in traffic, delayed at the airport, caught up at work, etc... This helps you decrease the chance of eating foods that are counterproductive and contrary to your new lifestyle.

EXHIBIT 4

Prayer and Word Study Consecration Chart

	Memorization & Word Study Appointment	Memorization & Word Study Attained	Prayer Appointment	Prayer Attained
Sunday				
Monday				
Tuesday				
Wednesday				
Thursday				
Friday				
Saturday				
WEEKLY TOTALS				

Prayer List:

SELF:

LOVED ONES:

OTHER:

EXHIBIT 5

Body Measurement Chart

	1st	2nd	3rd	4th	5th
Date:					
Weight:					
Calves	R L	R L	R L	R L	R L
Thighs	R L	R L	R L	R L	R L
Hips					
Glutes					
Lower Abdominals					
1" Above Navel					
Back and Chest					
Arms	R L	R L	R L	R L	R L
Shoulders					
Neck					
TOTAL:					

Disclaimer

The information, including opinions and recommendations, contained in this book and in the Faith & Fat Loss website are for educational purposes only and have not been evaluated by the FDA. Such information is not intended to be a substitute for medical advice, diagnosis, or treatment. No one should act upon any information provided in this book or in the Faith & Fat Loss website without first seeking medical advice from a qualified medial physician.

References:

www.biblegateway.com has been used for searching and referencing scripture from the King James Version Bible and other Bibles.

www.eliyah.com/lexicon.html has been used for searching scripture and researching the Greek and Hebrew definitions of the words in scripture.

www.wikipedia.com was used for references and definitions.

ACKNOWLEDGEMENTS

I want to express my deep gratitude to Sandra Lynn, who is not only my mother-in-law and friend, but has been with us through the whole process. I appreciate her intelligence and loving support as she has diligently edited and reviewed the pages of this book. It has been wonderful to witness the growth of her relationship with the Lord.

Thank you to Ryan Lindahl for his hard-work, professionalism, and creative touches in the layout of the book. It is a privilege and a rarity to work with someone whose standards are — excellence and efficiency.

To those of you who have prayed for us and this extraordinary book throughout the process – Thank you for your selfless commitment because we know that prayer makes a difference!! And a special thanks to Armando and Elva Herrera and Ted Belliston and Kim Rogers for their constant support and prayers.

We thank God for our ten children whom we love. Our prayer is that they would each have a passion and strong desire to live for the Lord and to make a difference in others lives.

Most of all we want to thank God for His love and patience, and for sending us Jesus Christ who is the answer to every dilemma that we could ever face. Thank you for choosing us to deliver this life-changing message to the world, and trusting that we would fulfill your will concerning this apostolic ministry.

Special Acknowledgement: I would like to thank God for my wife, Tonja, who truly loves the Lord and has a strong desire to do His will. I want to thank her for sitting down and intently listening to me, as I unveiled the vision that the Lord placed in my heart. She took this vision of faith, fat loss, and transformation on, as if it was her own, and we became one. Together we committed to each other and the Lord to fulfill the vision. I'm so proud of her spiritual growth throughout this time.

Tonja — I love you so much, and I look forward to every tomorrow because I get to spend it with you. Our precious relationship has been the best of my life. Not only are you my wife, but also my business partner, partner in ministry, my girlfriend, and truly my best friend.

ABOUT THE AUTHOR

Ron Williams is the author and developer of the Faith & Fat Loss Program and Book. Ron is one of the country's leading experts on exercise physiology, diet and nutrition, and fat loss. He has devoted his life to helping individuals physically, emotionally, and spiritually. Health problem's people experience from being overweight or obese has become his passion.

Ron Williams is one of the world's top natural athletes. Along with spiritual, intellectual, and academic experience, he is also one of the most decorated Natural Bodybuilders in the world. By applying his knowledge of Biblical principles in nutrition, fat loss, muscle development and body sculpting, Ron achieved the highest honor ever given in Natural Bodybuilding by becoming the sole recipient of the "Natural Bodybuilder of the Decade" award. Ron has won over 200 titles in the natural bodybuilding arena and holds seven Mr. Natural Universe titles, seven Natural Olympia titles, and seven Natural World titles. In November of 2008 he was inducted into the International Natural Bodybuilding Association's Hall of Fame.

As a professor of exercise physiology and nutrition, Ron was able to enhance many lives and teach his practical application of fat loss and body sculpting. He enjoyed his experience of teaching on a college level, but felt that the most important element was missing: the spiritual aspect. Using science and history to validate the Biblical principles found in scripture, Ron embarked on an in-depth study of diet and nutrition, with the word of God as a guide, and discovered timeless Biblical nutritional principles that would benefit all.

Ron is often called upon by organizations such as schools, athletic teams, corporations, and churches to give seminars, workshops, and conventions on exercise, the physiology of the body, diet and nutrition, and biblical and faith-based concepts. God has given him some tools that are easy to embrace, easy to understand, and easy to apply. Ron also has a training certification that equips Faith & Fat Loss ministers.

Ron has authored several books; including, "More than 21 Simple Ways to Lose Body Fat," and is the pastor of Back to the Foundation Church in Salt Lake City, Utah.

About Us

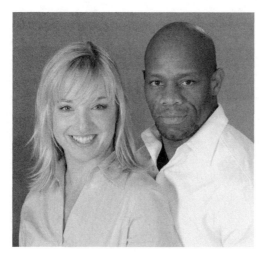

Ron and Tonja Williams brought together their diverse gifts to found Faith & Fat Loss in 2007. Ron brings 30 years of experience and vast knowledge in nutrition and physiology of the body, 19 years of ministry along with extensive fasting and prayer, and a God-given vision. As the spokesperson for Faith & Fat Loss, Ron has a unique ability to capture, connect, and minister to audiences. Tonja brings a creative ability to blend concepts and words together, along with 25 years of experience in business administration, ownership of a large corporation, and her God-given no nonsense approach to business. Because of her past successes, she is now the CEO of Faith & Fat Loss.

Ron and Tonja travel extensively teaching and preaching the Word of God bringing God's message of healing, health, wisdom, and salvation. The ministry's primary purpose is to minister healing to the wounded soul.

"Is anything worth more than your soul?" —**Mark 8:37 (NLT)**

For more information about Ron and Tonja or Faith & Fat Loss program and ministry, visit our website at: www.faithandfatloss.com. Or call 877-256-3488.